Super
Nutrition
for
Women

Super
Nutrition
for
Women

ANN LOUISE GITTLEMAN, Ph.D., C.N.S.
WITH J. LYNNE DODSON

BANTAM BOOKS

SUPER NUTRITION FOR WOMEN
A Bantam Book

PUBLISHING HISTORY
Bantam trade paperback edition published July 1991
Bantam revised edition / February 2004

Published by Bantam Dell
A Division of Random House, Inc.
New York, New York

LIBRARY OF CONGRESS CATALOGING-IN-PUBLICATION DATA
Gittleman, Ann Louise.
Super nutrition for women / Ann Louise Gittleman with
J. Lynne Dodson.— Rev. ed.
p.   cm.
Includes bibliographical references and index.
ISBN 0-553-38250-0
1. Women—Nutrition. 2. Women—Health and hygiene. I. Title.

RA778.G526 2004
613.2'082—dc22   2003058277

Manufactured in the United States of America
Published simultaneously in Canada

RRH 10 9 8 7 6 5 4 3 2

This book is lovingly dedicated to Edith and Arthur,
truly extraordinary human beings, who
also happen to be my parents

Acknowledgments

My deepest thanks and sincere appreciation go to the following extraordinary individuals who made this updated and revised edition possible:

To Caitlin Alexander, my insightful Bantam editor, who embraced a new *Super Nutrition for Women* so enthusiastically.

To Suzanne Cohn, my literary agent, who crossed the t's and dotted all the i's. Suzanne is a pleasure to know and work with on my projects.

To Linda Leekley, my editorial assistant and researcher par excellence, whose creative talents and attention to detail are top of the line. Linda is an angel!

To James, my super man, whose love and support make all things possible and worthwhile.

Contents

Super
Nutrition
for
Women

CHAPTER ONE

The Perils of Low-Fat Eating

Discovery consists in seeing what everybody else has
seen and thinking what nobody else has thought.
—ALBERT SZENT-GYORGI

Susan is 38 years old and she is dieting—again. She couldn't
count the number of diets she has been on since she first tried
to lose her "baby fat" at age 13. A half grapefruit for breakfast,
a salad with diet dressing for lunch, and broiled fish for dinner will help her reach her goal, she hopes. It seems to get
harder and harder each time. It takes less time to regain the
weight and more time to lose it, especially from around her
waist. Desserts are her downfall—she rewards her daytime
watchfulness with a "little treat" at night, Häagen-Dazs rum
raisin ice cream. Susan is a chronic dieter.

Twenty-eight-year-old Pat works at maintaining nutrition
despite a hectic lifestyle. She often reads articles on the latest
food trends and is quick to incorporate them into her diet.
Despite the latest "good fat" dietary trend, Pat is still overly
concerned about total fat and cholesterol. She avoids all oils,

butter, red meat, and eggs. She eats shredded wheat with skim milk and bananas for breakfast, stir-fried brown rice with vegetables and soy sauce for lunch, and pasta with meatless tomato sauce for dinner. Her one food vice is chocolate, which she craves, especially just before her period. Some of her friends call her a "nutrition buff."

At 18, Maryann is just beginning an independent life. One of the things she brought with her into her new apartment is her style of eating. Maryann is a "grabber"—a snacker who subsists on mini-meals as she rushes from one appointment to another. There are simply not enough hours in the day for her to sit down to three basic meals. Breakfast is a croissant and a cup of coffee, followed within a couple of hours by a diet cola and chips at her desk. Lunch with her coworkers is usually a hamburger, french fries, and a shake at a nearby fast-food chain. Dinner (if it's not pizza) has more variety thanks to the frozen-food section. Fruit-flavored yogurts are her favorite snack.

These three women have different eating habits but share some common complaints. They feel tired much of the time; they are irritable and often feel cold; they seldom sleep soundly through the night; they have various aches and pains that seem to have no cause; they are the first to get the season's colds; and vaginal infections, menstrual cramps, and bloating plague them every month. A visit to the doctor rules out a medical problem, so they think it must be "stress," "that time of life," "getting old," or "hormonal readjustment"—in any case, just something to live with. The longer they maintain their diet styles, the greater the likelihood that they will develop anemia, heart disease, cancer, osteoporosis, premenstrual syndrome, and arthritis.

Susan, Pat, and Maryann are fictionalized women, but they

represent the three basic female eating patterns I have observed while counseling thousands of clients both in person and on the Internet. I spotted these eating patterns repeatedly when I served as the nutrition director at the Pritikin Longevity Center in Santa Monica, California, and while working as a consultant to medical doctors, corporations, and environmental health clinics. By authoring twenty books on nutrition, I have worked to steer women away from these destructive patterns. In the last few years, it has been gratifying to help millions of women worldwide over the Internet via my interactive message board and my website, www.annlouise.com.

The chronic dieter, nutrition buff, and grabber are three basic female eating types I have noted over the past decades all over the country. These eating types have also been the focus of attention for USDA nutrition educators and other researchers throughout the country for decades, and they seem to cross economic and age categories. They can be identified in the diet histories of patients I counseled as far back as the early 1990s, spanning from Santa Fe to Washington, D.C., New York, Chicago, and San Francisco.

Whether in private practice, at hospitals, or in public health clinics, I have always required that my clients keep a food diary, recording what, when, and where they eat and drink, as well as their emotions at the time. By reviewing this record of total food intake over a period of three to seven days, I have been able to gauge their current eating habits.

Through my counseling I have evaluated the health impact of these eating styles and the concerns that have motivated women to adopt them in the first place. I have identified the potential health hazards of such eating patterns, and I have found food solutions that are nutritious, delicious, and convenient, whether at home or on the go.

CHRONIC DIETER

Let's begin with a little background on the chronic dieter who is dieting (again) for weight loss. A National Health Interview Survey found that almost half of American adult women were dieting at any one time.

In my own counseling experience, the majority of clients who have come to see me over the years have wanted to lose weight. Many had already tried the most popular diets of the day, including Weight Watchers, Slim•Fast, and Atkins. Were these women on the right track? The answer is yes and no. Based on conventional wisdom, there are basically only two ways to lose weight: burn more calories with exercise, or take in fewer calories with diet. Most women choose this second way.

Most of my clients tried to speed up the weight loss process by skipping meals, believing that by eating even less they would lose more weight faster.

As you read this, an estimated 124 million Americans are deliberately starving themselves in an effort to conform to society's and their own ideal body image. A large-scale survey in a popular women's magazine concluded that 75 percent of young women considered themselves too fat, even though 45 percent of them were actually underweight.[1] Twice as many women diet as men—and they are happier about losing weight than about any other success in their work or home lives. Even women who are underweight are trying to eat less. In fact, some health authorities believe only 20 percent of women eat normally, without dieting.

Yet the National Center for Health Statistics estimates that 47 percent of women over age 18 are overweight, with 20 percent being obese. A study by the Centers for Disease Control found that nearly 8 percent of women put on more than 30 pounds between the ages of 25 and 35. Over the past five decades, fatness has been increasing steadily in the United States. We spend a staggering $30 billion to $50 billion annually on diet books, pills, foods, and gimmicks, but at the same time we are consuming candy in record amounts. In the last 25 years, our consumption of soft drinks has increased by more than 114 percent, but we're eating only 10 percent more fruits and have upped our intake of vegetables by a scant 2 percent. Overall, Americans eat 15 percent less fat than they did a decade ago, but weigh 30 percent more.

I've often speculated that fatness is on the increase *because* of our preoccupation with dieting. Eating, not skipping meals, elevates the body's metabolic rate. In fact, as my former chronic dieters can testify, simply eating three meals a day can burn up to 10 percent more calories. This translates into 200 more burned calories for most women on a daily basis.

Taking in fewer calories usually means taking in fewer nutrients as well. A 1995 USDA study of food consumption found that women got significantly less than the recommended dietary reference intakes (DRIs) of seven nutrients: vitamins B_6 and E, calcium, magnesium, iron, folic acid, and zinc.

YO-YO DIETING RISKS

The effects of these schizophrenic eating habits have recently become the subject of serious research. At the University of Pennsylvania and elsewhere, scientists have studied what has become known as the yo-yo syndrome. Their conclusion— dieting can make you fat!

The yo-yo syndrome refers to cycles of weight gain and

loss from dieting. Unable to distinguish between famine and dieting, the body reacts to fewer calories with inherent defenses, biological mechanisms designed to withstand starvation and protect the species. Your basal metabolic rate actually slows down. Since this rate accounts for 60 to 75 percent of the energy used by the body—for routine functions like breathing and cell repair—its slowdown calls a halt to weight loss.

In addition, the body becomes more efficient in *storing* fat. Enzymes are complex proteins that regulate the body's chemical processes. One of them, called lipase, predigests dietary fat before it enters the intestine and thus makes the fat easier to digest and store. In yo-yo dieters, this enzyme becomes more active in preparing fat to be stored in fat cells.

These metabolic changes also cause a woman's body to gain weight faster and hold on to it once calorie intake returns to normal.

Kelly Brownell, Ph.D., and the researchers of the Weight Cycling Project have seen other hazards in yo-yo dieting in their preliminary data:

- Women who yo-yo diet may redistribute their body fat from the thighs and hips (the predominant location on the female body) to the abdomen. The fatter a person is from the waist up, the greater the risk for diabetes and heart disease.

- Yo-yo dieting may increase the body's ratio of fat to lean tissue. Women may lose considerable muscle tissue while dieting, but tend to regain it as fat.

- Yo-yo dieters may find their desire for fatty foods, many of which are unhealthful, increases.

- Additional risk from heart disease may come from the cycling of weight up and down. The long-term Framingham

Heart Study, which has monitored more than 5,000 people for over 50 years, has found that people who raised their body weight by 10 percent increased their risk of coronary artery disease by 30 percent. On the other hand, if they lost 10 percent of body weight, they decreased their risk by only 20 percent, for a net increase of 10 percent in risk every loss-gain cycle.

Now you can understand why every time you diet, it gets harder and harder to lose weight. It is not just common sense, but biochemical fact, that changing eating habits *gradually* (combined with exercise) is the only effective way to lose weight.

THE CHRONIC DIETER AND ENERGY-SAPPING DIETS

In addition to metabolic slowdown, diets that reduce calories also often exclude entire categories of foods. This sets women up for nutritional deficiencies. Red meat is a good case in point. A diet of fruits, vegetables, grains, and fish and poultry may be high in vitamins A and C and protein, but significantly deficient in blood-building iron, vitamin B_{12}, and the trace mineral zinc. These deficiencies can bring on anemia, asthma, hair loss, and psoriasis.

Women who feel deprived by low-calorie diets are more likely to cheat by devouring high-calorie, vitamin-deficient treats like gourmet cookies and rich desserts. How many times have I noted a coconut chocolate chip cookie, butternut ice cream, or a raspberry tart on the food diary of a chronic dieter who has sworn off red meat but treats herself to a fattening reward? These high-sugar foods may lead to anemia, osteoporosis, menstrual problems, and dry skin and hair by displacing more substantial foods in the diet.

THE NUTRITION BUFF

What about nutrition-conscious women like Pat? I have worked with hundreds of Pats, who make up the second largest group of patients consulting me for health problems. They think they are keeping fit and healthy by their watchfulness. Unfortunately, this is not the case for many of them.

Magazines and Internet sites that regularly poll their readers find that women say they are eating more poultry and fish, reading labels for nutrition information, and snacking on fruit.

Yet industry sales figures and national food consumption studies give a different view. Sadly, the 1995 USDA survey found no significant increase since 1977 in the percentage of women serving fish or fruits on a given survey day. As I pointed out earlier, the same study found women getting less than recommended amounts of vitamins B_6 and E, calcium, magnesium, iron, folic acid, and zinc, all critical to a woman's good health and optimum reproductive function.

FAT DECEPTION

For years, American women have been concerned about fats and, in particular, cholesterol. The late nutrition pioneer Nathan Pritikin, the American Heart Association, the Surgeon General, food editors all over the country, and even many food manufacturers urged a significant reduction of dietary fat as the way to health—*to 30 percent of calories*, down from the 40-plus percent most Americans consume. The Pritikin diet, with its emphasis on only 5 to 10 percent of calories from fats, convinced millions that fats were bad and linked with various degenerative diseases, particularly heart disease, America's number one killer.

The American public has been confused by a popular theory masquerading as absolute fact—a theory that has been told, retold, and told again over the past fifteen years. This theory—that fats are the ultimate dietary killers—has been extended to cover all fats, not just a few harmful ones. In my opinion, this has resulted in widespread harm to the overall health of our nation.

For so long, marketing by the nation's food companies has included phrases like "slash the fat," "reduced fat," and "fat free." The idea was that we could eat whatever we wanted, whenever we wanted, as long as the foods we ate were fat free. And many people, especially women, bought into this myth.

Women like Pat are still so anti-fat that they have not only sworn off every nut, seed, and avocado on the planet, but they'd rather be caught dead than use a drop of oil on their foods. Some of these women have become *too* lean from their obsessive dieting.

One of my clients, 33-year-old Gina, was a strong advocate of the low-fat, high-complex-carbohydrate diet because she believed it was the ideal diet for athletes. She ran almost five miles a day. When she consulted me because her periods had stopped, I explained that in addition to her extremely low-fat diet (fat makes hormones, as you will read later), her excessive exercise may have further reduced her body's fat stores and disrupted hormonal function, which ultimately reduced the circulating estrogen levels in her body. Overexercise causes the body to stop making estrogen and utilize calcium, which is estrogen dependent! I suggested that she decrease her running by one-half, to two and one-half miles a day, and that she gain at least five pounds. I also told her to add at least two tablespoons of olive oil to her daily diet. As it turned out, her period returned when she had regained only three pounds.

What advocates of the low-fat, high-carbohydrate diet overlooked was the evidence about the crucial—and positive—role some fats play in the diet. Women like Gina and others, who want to be thin but fertile, suffer the most from this nutritional one-sidedness.

But now other experts are finally beginning to agree with me about the importance of fats. As Gary Taubes reported in the New York Times in July 2002, "The dietary recommendations—eat less fat and more carbohydrates—may be the cause of the rampaging epidemic of obesity in America." Research points out "that there are plenty of reasons to suggest that the low-fat-is-good hypothesis has now effectively failed the test of time."[2]

As I will describe more fully in Chapter Three, certain vitamins must have fat present in order to be dissolved and absorbed into the body. Essential fatty acids (EFAs) play a positive role in a myriad of female reproductive disorders like premenstrual syndrome, viral and yeast infections, and infertility, as well as food allergy and immune disorders. EFAs strengthen cell membranes, which are our bodies' first defense against infections. Essential fats are also vital to healthy skin, hair, and nails (they are often added to hair and skin care products for topical application). Most important, essential fats are needed to form the hormonelike substances prostaglandins, which control the body's immune, cardiovascular, reproductive, and central nervous systems. Without prostaglandins (and the essential fats necessary for their production), our blood does not clot, tumors grow unchecked, cells become inflamed, and allergies rage out of control.

FAT AND CALCIUM

The right kind of fat is necessary for calcium availability in the soft tissues and to promote calcium elevation in the blood-stream so that muscles contract properly and maintain their tone, nerves function smoothly, blood clots when needed, and bones and teeth remain strong and healthy. Women who believe they are getting enough calcium through diet and supplements may be sabotaging themselves if they do not include enough of the right oils in their diets.

THE GRABBER VERSUS THE GRAZER

Eating a number of small meals each day can be an effective way to maintain a healthy weight and a stable blood sugar. This eating pattern is often called "grazing." However, Maryann, our mini-meal "grabber" and constant snacker, is fast becoming the norm in women's eating habits. Visit almost any major American shopping mall—shops selling chocolate chip cookies, European chocolates, croissants, and gourmet ice cream have joined the dress, shoe, and department stores as mall staples.

For many teenagers like Maryann, junk-food snacks and fast-food meals form a habit that is carried into adulthood. Fast-food restaurants make up almost 50 percent of all eating places in the United States, with more than 215,000 in operation. In fact, Americans spend more money on fast food than on movies, books, magazines, newspapers, videos, and music combined! Sadly, in the United States, more money is spent on calorie-laden fast food than on higher education.

Unlike sugar-laden junk food, which by definition has almost no food value, fast food does have some nutritional value. But it lacks several key vitamins and minerals—vitamins A, B_1, and C, and calcium, in particular—and a steady diet of fast food can be hazardous. The excesses of saturated fat, sodium, calories, and even sugar add to the problem.

The typical meal of hamburger, fries, and shake (not a milk shake, since it contains almost no milk) weighs in at almost 1,000 calories. Individuals who select the fish sandwich thinking it's healthier are in for a surprise—processing, breading, and deep-fat frying turn the wholesome fish into a high-calorie food filled with the wrong kind of fat.

COMPARISON OF TWO FAST-FOOD STAPLES

	Burger King Whopper	Burger King Big Fish
Calories	640	700
Protein	27 grams	26 grams
Carbohydrates	45 grams	56 grams
Fats	39 grams	41 grams
Sodium	870 milligrams	980 milligrams

Source: Adapted from *Fast Food Facts* by the Minnesota Attorney General's Office.

Women who eat on the run have created a booming market for convenience foods as well. Retail sales of frozen dinners and entrees were over $5.3 billion in 2000. Joining the three-course dinners are single-serving vegetable side dishes, gourmet entrees from around the world, and single-serving desserts.

Undeniably convenient and appealing, today's frozen foods achieve much of their appeal at the cost of healthfulness—the average frozen entree is over 50 percent nonessential fat, and some may contain over half of a woman's recommended daily sodium intake (1,100–3,300 milligrams), as this chart of just a few products highlights.

FROZEN DINNERS AND ENTREES
(AVERAGE OVER PRODUCT LINE)

Brand (serving size)	Fat (percent of cals)	Calories	Sodium (mg)
La Choy Dinners (12 oz)	10	243	1,822
Light & Elegant (9 oz)	19	259	880
Lean Cuisine (10 oz)	28	260	978
Weight Watchers (10 oz)	35	277	1,051
Armour Dinner Classics (11 oz)	39	391	1,339
Swanson 4-part Dinners (12 oz)	40	483	1,154
Le Menu (11 oz)	42	398	1,001
Budget Gourmet (10 oz)	43	373	849
Stouffer's Entrees (9 oz)	46	343	1,130
Old El Paso (na)	55	359	623

Source: © 1989 CSPI. Reprinted from *Nutrition Action Healthletter* (1875 Connecticut Ave., N.W., Suite 300, Washington, D.C. 20009-5728. $24.95 for 10 issues).

Maryann's problem as a grabber is related less to her pattern of eating than to what she eats. It is not necessary to eat three square meals a day to get the healthy balance of nutrients

and calories you need. Mini-meal eaters, or grazers, who select wisely benefit not only in good health but also in weight
control. In fact, a study reported in the *Journal of the American
Medical Association* found that women who ate one large meal a
day instead of several small ones were 25 times more likely to
store fat. The constant nibbling of the women who ate several
small meals stimulated their bodies' brown fat, a special fat-
burning tissue that produces body heat by burning calories
rather than storing the calories as fat cells. This meant that the
women's bodies stored less fat, their metabolism rose as their
food intake rose, and they lost weight.

I was first introduced to the concept of grazing (as opposed to grabbing) while working as the Director of Nutrition
at the Pritikin Longevity Center. In the early 1980s, the Center
served six mini-meals a day. This concept of constant feeding
was so integral to the program, but avant-garde at the time,
that the meals and food timings were printed on T-shirts,
which all the participants wore.

These mini-meals included many healthy foods, but they
lacked one key element—fat. Like the others on the program,
I was constantly grazing because I was always hungry. The fat-
free meals never left me satisfied. I can remember downing
bowl after bowl of oatmeal, wheat berries, or steamed barley
before my morning lectures in order to feel full. In fact, the
Pritikin fat-free regimen kept me from using even a bit of butter on my grains, so I was always hungry. (Fat slows down digestion; it takes at least two more hours for food to digest
with fat than without it. Hunger is therefore retarded when a
small amount of fat is added to the meals.) Thus, for fat-free
eaters, grazing was a necessity, almost an obsession.

Grazing is no longer considered avant-garde; it has become part of the current nutritional prescription of sound
dietary practice. If grazers choose wisely and include fats,

carbohydrates, and protein in balanced mini-meals, they can avoid the trap of becoming either a grabber or a Pritikin-style grazer.

THE SOUR SIDE OF SUGAR

All three eating styles share one potential pitfall—the lure of sugar in its many forms.

Desserts and sugar-laden snacks tempt a woman to choose happiness over health. Women who carefully monitor their food intake all day might indulge in a rich dessert reward at night—what one observer has termed the "Lean Cuisine/ Dove Bar mentality." Restaurants report an ever-increasing demand for the richest desserts they can produce. Nearly 40 percent of Americans eat ice cream often. In fact, Americans average 16 quarts per person per year. Gourmet brands, which are growing in popularity, get their richness from a recipe that is more than double the fat content of less expensive brands (a half cup of Häagen-Dazs vanilla ice cream contains 270 calories and 18 grams of fat; Breyers has 150 calories and 8 grams of fat).

These cravings are a complex mix of physiological and psychological factors, not yet fully understood. We know that fat in the diet gives a sense of fullness, so when the body is fat-starved, it sends insistent hunger messages. Good-tasting foods, including sweets, stimulate the palate and bring pleasure. There is a chemical basis for this in the mood-altering brain chemicals that are triggered by eating carbohydrates (cookies, cakes, muffins). In addition, many of us carry from childhood the "knowledge" that the reward for good behavior is a cookie, not a carrot.

Our sweet tooth contributes directly and indirectly to osteoporosis, premenstrual syndrome, excess weight, coronary artery disease, and cancer. Excess sugar is converted in the body to nonessential fatty acids (such as saturated fats) and cholesterol. One study by the USDA found that individuals who consumed 30 percent of their calories from sugar (slightly more than the typical American diet) developed significantly higher levels of cholesterol and triglycerides (fats) in their blood than did control subjects who had wheat starch substituted for the sugar.

Sugar consumption adversely affects the calcium-phosphorus balance so crucial to effective calcium absorption. If calcium levels in the blood are inadequate, calcium is drawn from bones and teeth, contributing to the development of osteoporosis and dental disease. Furthermore, calcium is essential for proper muscle function; deficiencies lead to muscle cramps, including those associated with menstruation. A recent American study has found that calcium also helps neutralize bile acids and fatty acids, which can irritate the bowel and contribute to the development of colon cancer.

Eating sugar with fat, as in ice cream, doughnuts and other baked goods, and butter-rich chocolates, causes the body to store fat more readily, rather than burning it for energy (see Chapter Four).

IS THERE A SOLUTION?

Many women are becoming more aware of how diet affects their bodies. They are making the connection between what they eat and how they feel. Many of my clients are eating some red meat, and more fish and vegetables. They're eating less salt and cutting back on their sugar habit. But this is only the beginning for the food-wise woman. We need to truly support female health. We need to know how chemical imbalances create a climate for disease and unhealthfulness. We must learn to protect the crucial "female minerals" from inhibitors—sugar, caffeine, soft drinks, and saturated fats—and to return valuable food staples to our diet, including lean red meat and eggs. We need to know the good side of cholesterol and dietary fats and learn to incorporate them into a balanced diet.

All of this can be done without exotic foods, chemistry books, obsessive concern for food, or, in most cases, nutritional supplements.

The suggestions I give in this book have worked for the thousands of women I have advised; they can work for you to restore the health and vitality you may have lost from chronic dieting, following the once popular low-fat and high-complex-carbohydrate diets, and eating fast food. I offer a nutritionally sound program to put the right fats, red meat, eggs, whole grains, and even fast foods in their proper place in your diet, to eliminate mineral inhibitors such as sugar and caffeine, and to banish the fear of fat—forever. It is my hope that this book will help you learn by firsthand experience that health is not a matter of chance, but a matter of choice.

CHAPTER TWO

Nutrition Notes for the Food-Wise Woman

Tell me what you eat and
I will tell you who you are.
—JEAN-ANTHELME BRILLAT-SAVARIN

BEFORE YOU BEGIN

Are you nourishing your body for the challenges you face daily? Are you a chronic dieter like Susan, a nutrition buff like Pat, or a grabber like Maryann? Or even a combination of all three? One way to help you understand your patterns of eating and food choices is to keep a food diary, recording your total intake of food and beverages for a specified period of time.

At the end of this chapter, you will find three copies of a food diary record sheet for you to record your total food intake for three consecutive days. The food diary asks you to record not only the food eaten, but the method of preparation: broiled, grilled, or fried, for example. If there is a sauce or dressing, remember to record it.

Unless you usually measure your portions, estimate the

amounts to the best of your ability using standard measurements, such as ¼ cup or 4 ounces.

When you eat (time of day) is included since it may give you clues to patterns of overeating and will help you plan mealtimes and snacks. Where you eat (setting) can be helpful to assess how frequently you eat at home, in restaurants, and in friends' homes, so you can better anticipate and plan for suitable food choices.

Finally, why you eat (emotions) should be recorded so that you can begin to distinguish between true biological hunger and "emotional hunger." The role of emotions in stimulating and controlling our eating behavior is the focus of considerable research. For example, Janet Polivy, Ph.D., professor of psychology and psychiatry at the University of Toronto, has found that when faced with stress or disappointment, women who diet are more likely to go off their diets and to eat more than women who aren't dieting. Emotional triggers are highly individual—some of us eat voraciously when we are in love, while others take our anger out on a plate of pasta or share our joy with a hot-fudge sundae. If you need to make changes in your eating patterns, noting these emotional triggers will be essential to success.

Include two workdays and one weekend day in keeping the food diary, to give you a more realistic picture of your overall pattern. Eat the way you ordinarily do, not the way you think you ought to for this record.

Once complete, your record becomes a valuable tool for putting the suggestions in this book to work. Look first at what you were eating and compare it against the following list of basics:

_____ 1 to 2 tablespoons of organic, cold expeller-pressed oil a day (include salad dressings and cooking oils: see Chapter Three for more on healthy oil)

_____ Five or more servings of fruits and vegetables each day (a serving is ½ cup cooked or 1 cup raw)

_____ Two or more servings of complex carbohydrates from grains, starchy vegetables, and legumes (½ cup equals one portion)

_____ At least two 4-ounce portions of protein three to four times per week (lean beef, skinless poultry, seafood, tofu, or tempeh)

_____ Up to two eggs per day

_____ At least two servings of a calcium source each day (such as 8 ounces of yogurt, a large stalk of broccoli, or even a calcium supplement, if you are simply unable to consume dairy products or enough calcium from foods)

_____ A daily source of cholesterol-lowering soluble fiber, such as ground or milled flaxseeds, an apple, a sweet potato, or a ½ cup of blood-sugar regulating kidney beans

Next, make note of how many of the following calcium or iron inhibitors you find.

_____ Coffee
_____ Soft drinks
_____ Sugar
_____ Tea
_____ Chocolate
_____ Aluminum

Finally, review your food diary for the social and emotional patterns that affect your eating habits. Are any of the following true for you?

_____ Eating is an important part of your social life.

_____ You eat when you have feelings of boredom, anger, or fatigue.

_____ Your reasons for eating at snacktime are different from those at mealtime.

_____ You snack at about the same time every day.

_____ Your eating patterns on the weekend differ from those on weekdays.

_____ Your largest meal is in the morning.

_____ Your largest meal is in the evening.

_____ You regularly skip one or more meals a day.

When you read my program, you will learn how to apply this information to the insights from your food diary to design the optimum plan for yourself. You can make better food choices and substitute foods that will cover areas in which you are deficient.

If your reasons for eating include depression, anxiety, boredom, tension, or fatigue, then your eating style is being controlled by emotional triggers rather than by hunger and nutritional need. Identifying these triggers is the first step in modifying your behavior.

If your social eating has an emotionally based component (a desire to be accepted or anxiety at new social settings), then anticipating these events can help you plan ahead for them. You will have a variety of choices for foods and beverages, all of which could enable you to fulfill any social needs without abandoning the plan. Chapter Eleven even has some suggestions for eating out within the plan.

Studies have shown that people who successfully changed their eating habits and food choices did so by making relatively modest changes in what, how much, and how often they ate. The less drastic the changes and the closer they matched the way the individuals normally ate and could eat in the future, the more successful these changes were.

So when you complete your review and begin your plan for change, be realistic and decide on small, concrete steps. For example, if you find that you are most apt to grab junk food in the midafternoon when hunger pangs strike, plan ahead and keep fresh fruit handy. If you find that you tend to skip breakfast and lunch and overeat at dinner, make an effort to eat something in the morning and early afternoon—even a hard-boiled egg or a fruit shake. If fiber is your deficiency but you hate oat bran cereals, then get your fiber from beans or raw fruits or vegetables.

You will find that the menu plans and recipes in Chapter Twelve do not generally include exotic ingredients; in many cases, they represent a stepping-off point, a halfway measure to move you toward long-term health and well-being.

THE NUTRITION NOTES

You have decided—you choose health. You want to feel better, look better, and live better now and in the future. This section summarizes my approach, developed through counseling thousands of women and described in greater detail in following chapters, to help you achieve this goal.

- **Don't be a yo-yo.** The yo-yo diet syndrome (the lose, gain, and regain cycles) can be more hazardous to health than remaining overweight. Very low calorie diets, particularly when combined with exercise, can drastically lower metabolic rate. Chronic dieters can regain more fat faster with regained fat redistributed around the abdominal area, which increases the risk of diabetes and heart disease. The ratio of fat to lean protein also increases with constant dieting, and the risk of heart disease can rise as much as 30 percent.

  By putting essential fats in your diet and following the other notes outlined here, you will lose weight without crash dieting.

- **Optimize calcium intake.** As I stress in Chapter Eight, choose high-quality calcium foods. Full-fat and low-fat dairy products, including yogurts, low-fat cottage cheese, and part-skim cheeses, are among the most concentrated calcium sources. You can get calcium from other sources as well, especially if you are allergic to dairy products. These include leafy green vegetables like broccoli, bok choy, kale, and collard greens. Sea vegetables like hijiki (popular in Japanese cuisine) contain 14 times the calcium of a glass of milk. Wakame provides 1,300 milligrams of calcium in a little less than ½ cup, while kombu provides 800 milligrams in the same sized portion.

  Take full advantage of the calcium you do get by eliminating the inhibitors: soft drinks, cocoa, coffee, tea, aluminum, and excessive grain intake. The phosphoric acid in soft drinks (regular and diet), the phytic acid in grains, and the caffeine in chocolate, coffee, and tea all interfere with calcium absorption or increase its excretion. Aluminum from pots and pans, cans, antacids, baking powders, and even tap water leaches calcium from your body.

- **Engage in weight-bearing exercise.** Research has shown that such exercise helps retain calcium in your bones. If you want to burn fat in the process, try to maintain continuous movement for 45–60 minutes daily. Brisk walking, cycling, rowing, swimming, or rebounding on a mini-trampoline are the best exercises to burn fat calories. Activities like calisthenics, volleyball, racquetball, and tennis, which feature stop-and-start movements, are best to burn carbohydrates. The most efficient fat burning occurs when you exercise before a meal, not after, so that digestion is not impacted.

- **Beef up blood-building iron.** Consume at least two servings (4 ounces each) of lean beef weekly and include iron-rich legumes and green, leafy vegetables in your diet. Vegetarians should emphasize iron-rich beets and can consider herbal supplements like yellow dock and dandelion root for easily assimilable iron. A good vitamin C source, like citrus fruits, tomatoes, or a baked potato, eaten with the iron-rich food further enhances iron absorption. Cooking in cast-iron pots contributes small amounts of vital iron to foods.

- **Include eggs and beef.** There are other reasons, besides your need for extra iron, to include beef in your regular diet, as I discuss in Chapter Four. It is a valuable source of zinc; the stearic acid it contains may actually lower serum cholesterol levels. Eggs contain the richest source of the sulfur-bearing amino acid L-cysteine, so important for skin, hair, and nail health. Choose eggs that are labeled high in omega-3s. Eating eggs rich in omega-3 fatty acids has also been found to reduce the risk of heart disease, depression, and Alzheimer's disease. Both eggs and beef are low-calorie, economical sources of protein, manganese, and other essential minerals. Up to 2 eggs per day, including those used in baking, and at least two 4-ounce servings of red meat weekly are recommended in my plan.

- **Put fats in their place.** Include 2 tablespoons of healthy fat every day in salad dressings and cooking.

    Eliminate all sources of damaged fats, such as commercial vegetable oils, hydrogenated oil products (margarine and vegetable shortening), and all products containing them. Use only organic, cold expeller-pressed oils.

    Unless you are among the 10 percent who have been diagnosed with high cholesterol levels (total cholesterol level above 200 mg/dl, for example), you should not need to pay special attention to cholesterol if you are eating essential fats and following the other recommendations.

- **Control your sweet tooth.** Avoid simple sugars, sweeteners, and refined carbohydrates. Keep your fruit consumption to three to five portions a day, preferably the fruit itself rather than juice. A portion is 1 small banana, 12 cherries, 1 small apple, or ½ grapefruit; for more details, see Chapter Ten. Both refined sugar and natural sugar products (even fruit and fruit juice) can play havoc with your energy levels and contribute to high blood levels of triglycerides. Sugar can cut calcium absorption and encourage yeast overgrowth, contributing to fatigue and a variety of allergic and mental symptoms. Excess sugar can also block the manufacture of beneficial prostaglandins from essential fatty acids.

- **Vary complex carbohydrates.** Choose more legumes and vegetables such as potatoes, squash, peas, and root vegetables. By diversifying your diet, you avoid gluten intolerance from overdoing consumption of grains like wheat, rye, oats, and barley; the phytic acid that inhibits calcium absorption; and the excess carbohydrates that may feed yeast infections.

• **Value multicolored vegetables daily and weekly.** Eating a rainbow of vegetables contributes fiber, vitamins, minerals, and phytonutrients for all-around health. Feature cruciferous vegetables like Brussels sprouts, cabbage, broccoli, cauliflower, rutabagas, and turnips at least twice a week to help reduce the risk of cancer. Eat dark green, yellow, or orange vegetables at least three or four times per week. Dark green leafy vegetables are rich in antioxidants and lutein, which help neutralize the free radicals that damage cells. Yellowish orange vegetables are packed with flavonoids and carotenoids, which contain alpha-carotene, beta-carotene, lutein, and lycopene to further help suppress cancer risk. Carotenoids—such as lycopene, a red pigment found in tomatoes—are also known to reduce the chance of developing lung and stomach cancer.

• **Fiber up your diet.** The average American eats approximately 11 grams of fiber per day, yet the National Cancer Institute suggests between 25 and 35 grams to help prevent colon and rectal cancer. Choose a balance of water-soluble fibers from ground flaxseeds, oats, legumes, sweet potatoes, and other fresh fruits and vegetables to control cholesterol and even out blood sugar levels.

• **Avoid too much salt.** Excess salt contributes to high blood pressure and fluid retention and bloating. Many canned, frozen, bottled, and packaged foods contain hidden salt, so become a label reader. Avoid soy sauce, tamari, and salt added to foods at the table. Aim for an average daily intake of

1,500 milligrams, the equivalent of ¾ teaspoon. Remember that many foods are naturally high in sodium, including carrots, celery, and beets. Eating a well-balanced diet, without ever using a salt shaker, will give you all the sodium you need for good health.

- **Cook for health.** Choose healthy cooking methods for your healthy foods. Baking, roasting, broiling, poaching, and steaming are best for daily cooking. Frying, charcoal grilling, and smoking should be limited because of the harmful chemicals they produce in food.

- **Avoid aluminum.** Do not use aluminum or foil for cooking, reheating, or wrapping foods. This pliable heavy metal leaches into acidic foods and accumulates in the kidneys, brain, and intestines. It interferes with the body's ability to absorb and process calcium through chemical interaction with other minerals.

- **Optimize magnesium intake.** Magnesium is a highly underrated mineral, often overshadowed by its cousin calcium. As a natural, safe calcium-channel blocker, magnesium protects against heart disease. It also helps prevent osteoporosis, regulates nerve cell function, keeps the bowels working properly, and promotes sleep. A magnesium deficiency can cause high blood pressure, muscle cramps, depression, fatigue, learning disabilities, and an irregular heartbeat. In fact, getting enough magnesium can correct a wide variety of health problems.

FOOD DIARY

Day of the week _____

WHAT (Name of food/preparation)	AMOUNT (Portion size)	WHEN (Time of day)	WHERE (Setting)	WHY (Emotions)
Meal one				
Meal two				
Meal three				
Snacks				

FOOD DIARY

Day of the week _____

WHAT (Name of food/preparation)	AMOUNT (Portion size)	WHEN (Time of day)	WHERE (Setting)	WHY (Emotions)
Meal one				
Meal two				
Meal three				
Snacks				

FOOD DIARY

Day of the week _____

WHAT (Name of food/preparation)	AMOUNT (Portion size)	WHEN (Time of day)	WHERE (Setting)	WHY (Emotions)
Meal one				
Meal two				
Meal three				
Snacks				

CHAPTER THREE

The Case Against Fat-Free, High-Grain Diets

Each progressive spirit is opposed by a thousand mediocre minds appointed to guard the past.

—MAURICE MAETERLINCK

Surprisingly, there are many health-conscious women like Pat and Gina who are still following the antiquated dietary model of the 1980s and 1990s—a no-fat, high-complex-carbohydrate diet. What they need to understand is that their fat-free, predominantly grain-based foods may actually be creating many of the health problems women face today in the 21st century. Women are eating their way into hormonal dysfunction.

Way back in 1974, when Nathan Pritikin published his book *Live Longer Now*, he struck a responsive chord for many Americans. The American Heart Association was urging us to cut back on fat consumption, and the death rate from cardiovascular disease was continuing its steady rise.

Although he was not a physician, Pritikin had reviewed countless pieces of research over a 25-year period. When he was diagnosed in 1955 with a severe heart condition, he began reviewing medical literature on the degenerative diseases of the Western world, such as cardiovascular disease, high blood pressure, diabetes, and cancer. He came to the landmark con- clusion that the fat in our diet was the culprit. He believed that by severely reducing our fat intake to just 5–10 percent of calories and increasing complex carbohydrates to 80 percent, we could achieve the lower rates of degenerative diseases seen in native cultures like the Bantus of South Africa and the Tarahumara Indians of Mexico.

This was a spartan diet, and Pritikin was criticized by the American Heart Association, the American Diabetes Association, and many physicians. Yet he persisted. He established Pritikin Longevity Centers in California, Florida, and Pennsylvania. A few years after his death in 1985, most experts and profes- sional organizations all over the country had moved toward his recommendations, including many of those who had pre- viously criticized him.

CONCERN OVER NO-FAT

Thankfully, my early concerns over low-fat diets have been mirrored by other health professionals. This has given rise to the popularity in the late 1990s and today of lower-carb, higher-fat diets. For example, Dr. Barry Sears came on board and conveyed a nutritional philosophy similar to my own when he created the Zone Diet. For ten years, I often felt like the lone proponent of the importance of dietary fats. So it is gratifying that other professionals have now joined with me to educate the public on this important health issue. But how did this transformation come about?

It was clear to me years ago that something was not quite

right. The Pritikin diet and others like it did not prove to be the miracle we sought. I saw it in the participants I worked with as Nutrition Director of the Pritikin Longevity Center in Santa Monica and later in private practice: women who should have felt good and looked good on their low-fat, high-carbohydrate diet were instead tired, cold, retaining fluids, and experiencing menstrual difficulties and recurring yeast infections. Their diet records revealed they were hungry most of the time and tried to raise their energy levels with sugar-laden cookies, fruit juices, and frozen yogurt. Their hair and skin were dry, their nails brittle and ridged. Many had stopped menstruating.

The factor of the ridged nails, which I recounted in my first book, *Beyond Pritikin*, created quite a stir among my readers. I have received countless letters from readers all over the country who reported seeing ridges develop on their nails after being on a low-fat, high-complex-carbohydrate diet for several months. As I explained in *Beyond Pritikin*, this condition is a sign of a vitamin or mineral deficiency, which may be due to the high levels of fiber that take essential minerals like calcium and iron out of the body. Any diet that is not good for the hair, skin, and nails is not good for the rest of your body either.

Other experts also had doubts. If fats were the answer to Americans' high rate of degenerative diseases, how were the researchers to explain:

- The Eskimos, who are virtually free of cardiovascular disease despite a diet that is 70 percent fat
- The Greeks and Italians along the Mediterranean, with a death rate from heart disease half that of Americans, yet with a diet of 40 percent fat (a percentage comparable to that of the typical American diet)

• The Masai tribe of East Africa, living on a diet consisting almost entirely of meat and milk, who show low blood cholesterol levels and negligible heart disease

• The results of an 11-year study of residents of Roseto, Pennsylvania, who consume high-cholesterol and high-fat foods, which showed blood cholesterol levels averaging 224 (average for the nation) and almost no heart attacks in men under 55

What we've learned is that fats are generally misunderstood and unduly maligned. Not only are some fats good, but the essential fatty acids (omega-3 and the "good" omega-6s) are vital to the integrity of the body's cell membranes and to the maintenance of the cardiovascular, immune, reproductive, and central nervous systems. These fats, along with their far-reaching health benefits, are the ones most likely to be deficient in a woman's diet.

HOW FATS ARE CLASSIFIED

Let's talk briefly about how fats are defined. All fatty acids are classified as saturated, monounsaturated, or polyunsaturated. (These terms relate to the type and number of hydrogen bonds in the chemical structure of the fatty acid.) Their structure affects the movement of the molecules and the susceptibility of the fat to heat and oxidation.

All fats are a blend of the three types, but one type predominates, giving the fat its status as a saturate, monounsaturate, or polyunsaturate. Major food sources of each fat group are listed below.

Saturates—*Animal sources:* pork, lamb, and beef fats (lard, tallow, suet); organ meats; full-fat dairy products such as whole milk, cream cheese, ice cream, and butter. *Vegetable sources:* coconut oil, cocoa butter, palm oil, and palm-kernel oil.

Monounsaturates—*Vegetable, legume, and seed sources:* olive, macadamia, avocado, almond, apricot kernel, peanut, high-oleic safflower and sunflower oils, and rice bran oil.

Polyunsaturates—(omega-3) *Animal sources:* marine oils from salmon, mackerel, herring, cod, sardines, rainbow trout, shrimp, oysters, halibut, tuna, sablefish, bass, flounder, and anchovies; cold-water fish such as trout and crappie. *Vegetable sources:* flaxseed oil, perilla oil, hemp, pumpkin seeds, soybeans, walnuts, wheat germ, wheat sprouts, fresh sea vegetables, leafy greens, and purslane.

Polyunsaturates—(omega-6) *Animal sources:* mother's milk, organ meats, lean meats. *Vegetable sources:* safflower, sunflower, corn, soy, sesame, hemp, raw nuts and seeds, legumes, spirulina, leafy greens. *Botanicals:* borage, evening primrose oil, and black currant seed oil.

PERCENTAGE OF FATTY ACIDS BY SATURATION TYPE IN VARIOUS OILS

Type of Oil	Saturated	Monounsaturated	Polyunsaturated
Almond	9	65	26
Apricot kernel	6	63	31
Avocado	20	70	10
Coconut	92	6	2
Corn	17	29	54
High-oleic safflower*	8	75	17

Type of Oil	Saturated	Monounsaturated	Polyunsaturated
High-oleic sunflower*	8	81	11
Macadamia	12	85	3
Olive	10	82	8
Palm kernel	83	16	1
Peanut	13	60	27
Safflower	8	13	79
Sesame	13	46	41
Soy	14	28	58
Sunflower	8	26	66

Source: Adapted from Spectrum Naturals, Petaluma, CA.

* High-oleic oils are produced from a new breed of sunflower and saf-flower seed, which contains higher levels of the monounsaturated fatty acid, oleic acid.

SATURATED FATS

Saturated fats have been labeled the bad guys in the American diet because they have been connected with high cholesterol and hardening of the arteries. However, Dr. Mary Enig, a well-respected researcher in the field of fats and oils, has stated that "the idea that saturated fats cause heart disease is completely wrong. However, the statement has been 'published' so many times over the last three or more decades that it is very difficult to convince people otherwise."[1]

In her book *Know Your Fats: The Complete Primer for Understanding the Nutrition of Fats, Oils, and Cholesterol*, Dr. Enig offers outstanding research that tells the true tale of how important fats are and which ones actually cause problems. She zeroes in on the real culprits—hydrogenated and partially hydrogenated vegetable fats and oils, with their troublemaking trans fatty acids—and cites them as the catalysts behind many of our health problems. Consuming trans fatty acids produces many adverse effects, such as:

- Lowering HDL ("good" cholesterol)
- Raising LDL ("bad" cholesterol)
- Raising total serum cholesterol levels 20 to 30 percent
- Lowering the milk volume in lactating females
- Increasing blood insulin levels, upping the risk for diabetes
- Escalating the adverse effects of essential fatty acid deficiency
- Potentiating the formation of free radicals (those unstable molecules of oxygen associated with aging and degenerative disease)

As you can see, the real villains causing our health problems may well be vegetable fats in the form of processed vegetable oils, margarine, vegetable shortenings, and baked goods made from these products. So, remember, the only real problem with saturated fats is that they are often eaten in excess and act as metabolic roadblocks in the metabolism of the essential fatty acids. Saturated fats are found in many of our most popular foods, including full-fat dairy products such as cheese and ice cream, as well as in tropical vegetable oils such as palm, palm kernel, and coconut oils, used in many baked goods. Cookies, candies, cakes, crackers, and cereals often contain one or more of these highly saturated vegetable oils. Known as the tropical fats, they are high in the easily digested medium chain fats that are more likely to be utilized as fuel rather than stored as fat by the body. As long as the saturates are kept in balance with our intake of the omega-3 and "good" omega-6 essential fatty acids, they are much more healthy than the trans fat substitutes such as vegetable shortening.

The good news is that meat is healthier than previously believed. A landmark study in the New England Journal of Medicine found that the stearic acid component in beef fat may be helpful in lowering cholesterol and in moderating other fats in the diet. So if you are concerned about saturated fats, you do not have to eliminate red meat completely—simply choose lean cuts such as the tip or eye of the round and top round, which rate close to chicken in levels of fats and calories but contain more minerals.

MONOUNSATURATED FATS

My favorite all-purpose monounsaturated oil is called MacNut Oil and it comes from macadamia nuts. Macadamia oil (available in health food stores and via the Internet at MacNut.com) contains high amounts of naturally occurring antioxidants, and is the oil highest in monounsaturated fats (85 percent monounsaturates versus 82 percent in olive oil). It can be used in salad dressings, for baking, and for cooking, with no danger of being transformed into deadly trans fatty acids. MacNut Oil is created using a proprietary process of pressing the nuts using a chilled expeller press and then filtering the oil. This light, buttery monounsaturated fat has the ideal ratio (1:1) of omega-3 to omega-6 fatty acids.

Many years ago research by Scott M. Grundy, M.D., director of the University of Texas Health Sciences Center, highlighted the special benefit of monounsaturated fats. In the New England Journal of Medicine, March 1986, Dr. Grundy reported that monounsaturates lowered total blood cholesterol levels even more than a low-fat, high-carbohydrate diet did. Perhaps more important, the monounsaturate high-oleic safflower oil selectively lowered the "bad" cholesterol and left more of the "good" cholesterol than did the polyunsaturate safflower oil (more about cholesterol in Chapter Four).

POLYUNSATURATED FATS: THE ESSENTIAL FATTY ACIDS

There are 46 essential nutrients that are critical for total body function. These include 20 minerals, 15 vitamins, 9 amino acids (the building blocks of protein), and 2 fatty acids (the building blocks of fat). These nutrients cannot be made from other substances; we must get them in the natural state from foods or, in some cases, dietary supplements.

We need a balance of the proper essential fats from both the omega-3's and omega-6's. These two groups of polyunsaturated fatty acids are essential for the regulation of every function in the human body. From the original omega-3 fatty acid, alpha-linolenic acid, our bodies make eicosapentaenoic acid (EPA) and docosahexaenoic acid (DHA). From the original omega-6 fatty acid, linoleic acid, our bodies produce gamma-linoleic acid (GLA). These two series of essential fatty acids are found naturally in omega-3-rich cold-water fish and omega-6-rich unprocessed vegetable, seed, and botanical oils. Both groups must be provided by the diet because the body cannot produce them itself.

These essential fatty acids (EFAs) must be present in the diet along with vitamin E and the B vitamins to produce sex and adrenal hormones and control cell growth. The benefits

credited to polyunsaturates are actually the health benefits
provided by the essential fatty acids.

For example, the EFAs are a component of the outer membrane of every cell, where they protect against invading viruses,
bacteria, and allergens. Flexibility and fluidity of the cell membrane depend on the presence of the EFAs. EFAs increase metabolism and energy production. They help dissolve body fat into
body fluids (yes, eat fat to lose fat!), decreasing blood cholesterol
and triglyceride levels. They distribute the fat-soluble vitamins A,
D, E, and K throughout the body, help insulate the nerves, and
have a role in maintaining a steady body temperature.

Essential fatty acids are also the building blocks from which
prostaglandins are made. These hormonelike substances regulate every organ, tissue, and cell in the human body at a basic
cellular level.

Research continues on the exact roles of the three main types
of prostaglandins and their many subgroups. What is known,
however, is that they strengthen immunity, regulate sodium excretion, stimulate hormone production, contract intestinal muscles, and regulate blood clotting. One type stimulates production
of thyroid hormone, ensuring the energy we need. Decreased
levels of prostaglandins may bring on some types of asthma; researchers know that if levels are adequate, muscles in the lungs
relax and blood flow increases. Prostaglandins have proven helpful in relieving various symptoms of premenstrual syndrome
(PMS) as well as depression and conditions ranging from arthritis and ulcers to migraines and cancer.

The specific essential fatty acids needed for prostaglandin
production are alpha-linolenic acid and cis-linoleic acid. In
brief, the process is:

1. Alpha-linolenic acid (from the omega-3 family of fatty
   acids) is converted to eicosapentaenoic acid (EPA). Helping

with this conversion are vitamin B_6, magnesium, zinc, insulin, and an enzyme.

2. EPA is converted to the prostaglandin E3 (PGE3).

The chemical conversion process for the omega-6 fatty acid, cis-linoleic acid, is very similar:

1. Cis-linoleic acid is converted to gamma-linoleic acid (GLA), again with the help of vitamin B_6, magnesium, zinc, insulin, and an enzyme.

2. GLA undergoes a chemical change to produce prostaglandin E1 (PGE1), aided by vitamins B_3 and C.

3. Alternatively, GLA can be converted to arachidonic acid through the action of another enzyme.

4. Arachidonic acid is then converted to prostaglandin E2 (PGE2).

The best sources of cis-linoleic acid are oils that are 100 percent expeller-pressed and unrefined. These oils are produced not with solvents or chemicals but by pressing the raw material (sesame seeds, olives, etc.) through a screw press at the lowest possible temperature to release the oils. Unlike refined oils, an unrefined oil is not filtered a second time, bleached, or deodorized; it retains more of the nutrients of the source material.

Since cis-linoleic acid is converted to GLA before the ultimate production of prostaglandins, you can also sustain this process by using some of the plants and oils that contain GLA itself: borage, spirulina (a type of plankton), evening primrose oil, and black currant seed oil.

The omega-3 alpha-linolenic acid is found in wheat sprouts,

wheat germ, and nuts and seeds (and their oils) including walnuts, flaxseed, and soybeans. The direct form of EPA is found in high amounts in oil from cold-water fatty fish such as sardines, salmon, and mackerel. It is more potent in the fresh varieties and can deteriorate quickly in the freezing or canning process.

Commercially processed oils, hydrogenated margarines, and fried foods—what I call damaged fats—interfere with the transformation of GLA and EPA into prostaglandins. During processing the beneficial polyunsaturates are exposed to excess heat, air, light, or hydrogenation, making them unusable for the human body.

There are several other factors that hamper prostaglandin production by blocking the enzyme that transforms cis-linoleic acid into GLA. These factors include saturated fats, cholesterol, aging, alcohol, high blood sugar, viral infection, radiation, and aspirin. Thus, many individuals may have difficulty in obtaining the proper expeller-pressed unrefined oils in the first place, while others have difficulty in converting EFAs into prostaglandins because of dietary, illness, medication, and life-style factors.

CLA: The New Kid on the Block

Recent groundbreaking research on the omega-6's has focused upon conjugated linoleic acid (CLA), making CLA the most popular new kid on the block. Exhaustively studied since its discovery over a decade ago, CLA has demonstrated an ability to help on many health fronts. Researchers from the University of Wisconsin believe that we are getting no CLA from the foods we eat today due to two major factors. The first factor is the fat-is-bad mind-set that is only now beginning to dissipate and that has steered Americans away from the only possible CLA dietary sources available—beef, lamb, and full-fat dairy products like cheese, milk, and butter. The second factor is that livestock is no longer grass-fed but instead is raised in feedlots on grain, which decreases the animals' levels of CLA by nearly 80 percent. Thus, even people who consume animal protein are missing out on this important nutrient. For most of my clients, I recommend a daily dose of 1,000 milligrams three times per day.

Laboratory research over the past twenty years has shown that CLA reduces the body's ability to store fat for energy by controlling the enzymes that release fat from the cells into the bloodstream. Lack of this critical fatty acid in the American diet is definitely a contributing factor to the steady rise in obesity over the past thirty years, even though we have reduced our overall fat intake.

A year-long U.S. clinical trial led by Dr. Richard Atkinson, the president of the American Obesity Association, was completed in 1999. Atkinson's study was designed to determine the effects of CLA on body composition in obese men and women. The study followed 80 people as they dieted and then regained weight. The results showed that those who took CLA put the pounds back on in a ratio of half fat to half muscle— an extraordinary finding considering that most regained pounds are usually redeposited as 75 percent fat and 25 percent muscle.[2] Today, there are more than 100 studies being conducted on this previously unrecognized nutrient.

THE FAT–WEIGHT LOSS CONNECTION

Eating the right fat will also help you achieve balanced weight loss. GLA has been found to stimulate the brown fat of the body. Thanks to the pioneering research of Dr. George Bray, the leading American expert on brown fat, we now know that brown fat is a special fat-burning tissue that burns and dissipates excess calories for heat, rather than depositing them for storage as fat. Unlike white fat, which is the insulating layer on the outside of the body, brown fat lies deeper, surrounding organs such as the heart, kidneys, and adrenals. Researchers have hypothesized that thin people may have activated brown fat, while overweight individuals may have dormant brown fat. It takes a certain type of dietary fat to activate the body brown fat. GLA, one of the EFAs we have been discussing, found directly in borage and evening primrose oil or in the preliminary form in safflower oil, stimulates brown fat metabolism.

In fact, thousands of women have expressed their amazement on my Web site. By following my Fat Flush® eating plan—which puts the right kinds of fats back into their diets—they have flushed away the pounds and dropped dress sizes. And they are keeping the weight off! During the Lifestyle phase, they consume 1 tablespoon of flaxseed oil, 360 milligrams of GLA, and 3,000 milligrams of CLA. As a result, they have lost their fear of fat and gained healthy and more beautiful bodies.

THE FAT–YEAST CONNECTION

Essential fatty acids, especially in the omega-3 group, slow down the growth of yeast organisms in the body. Yeast overgrowth is thought to affect as many as one in three Americans. Overgrowth of *Candida albicans*, common in women, causes symptoms ranging from allergies to throat infections to joint swelling to memory loss, and repeated vaginal or bladder infections. The EFAs stimulate the process of oxidation, which spells death to the oxygen-hating (anaerobic) yeast.

Healthy skin, hair, and nails owe much to the EFAs. EFAs plump up the cell membranes and help repair old membranes and construct new ones. Eczema, psoriasis, dandruff, hair loss, dryness, and brittle nails respond to added EFAs in the diet.

By helping to control the flow of body oils, EFAs regulate the skin's metabolism and counter thick, dry skin from the inside out. Healthy collagen is also a benefit from the EFAs. The beautifying skin vitamins A and E must be dissolved in fat to be used within the body to provide glowing skin and hair.

Carrying vitamin D as well as calcium into the soft tissues, EFAs help protect against osteoporosis since calcium must have vitamin D present for absorption. Depletion of calcium from bones leads to brittleness.

OTHER CARBOHYDRATE-RELATED DISORDERS

A low-fat, high-carbohydrate diet causes problems because it doesn't include adequate essential fat, but it causes an equal number of problems by emphasizing carbohydrates, in the form of excessive grains.

The popularity of low-fat, high-carbohydrate diets is just one factor in the phenomenal rise in grain consumption over the past 25 years, especially wheat, which represents over 80 percent of our total grain consumption. Wheat flour consumption has risen from 110 pounds per person in 1972 to 150 pounds today.

According to Beatrice Trum Hunter, food editor of *Consumers' Research Magazine* and author of *Gluten Intolerance*:

- Present-day food technology relies heavily on wheat—as emulsifiers, stabilizers, and food starches in such varied foods as ice cream, catsup, and some instant coffees.

- The growth of vegetarianism spurred many new ways to serve grains.

- The "gentrification" of pasta changed it from a food for the poor or a food that was considered "fattening" to a gourmet food item capable of being dressed up or down.

- Urged to increase fiber intake, we have expanded our consumption of cereals, meals, and flours.

- Interest in ethnic cuisines, many of which include more grains than does standard American fare, has also played a part.

Grains are relative newcomers in the human diet—it has been only about 10,000 years since the development of agriculture. As an article in the *New England Journal of Medicine* points out, our prehistoric ancestors ate raw vegetables and low-fat meats with occasional seasonal fruits and nuts and seeds. They did not eat grains or dairy products.

Our digestive system has changed very little since then, but our diets have changed significantly. The excessive intake of carbohydrates creates fertile ground for a number of health problems, including gluten intolerance, insulin resistance, metabolic syndrome, and diabetes.

Many of these problems with carbohydrates actually stem from a component of many grains, called gluten. Gluten consists of the two protein substances glutenin and gliadin. Gliadin seems to be the problem in sensitive individuals.

Symptoms of gluten intolerance (also known as celiac disease, sprue, or gluten-induced enteropathy) were described almost 2,000 years ago. Once rare, these symptoms are now increasing, affecting 1 of every 133 Americans. They include diarrhea, anemia, muscle spasms and cramps, bone or joint pain, headache, bloating, and intestinal pain.

There appears to be a genetic predisposition, but diet is the initiating factor. The gluten damages the intestinal lining, which then does not properly absorb the products of digestion. Minerals, vitamins, proteins, and fats pass out of the body, unused. Loss of vitamin D, calcium, and phosphorus brings on bone changes and muscle cramps. Loss of vitamin B_{12} and folic acid may bring on pernicious anemia; loss of iron can create iron deficiency anemia.

The high fiber content of gluten-rich grains (wheat, rye, oats, and barley), taken in excess, can help remove valuable nutrients such as zinc, calcium, and iron from the body before they can be absorbed and used. Both zinc and calcium are necessary for the release of insulin from the pancreas to metabolize sugar and other carbohydrates.

Insulin resistance affects nearly 75 million Americans, and some experts believe that it is the cause for at least half of all heart attacks. This condition may be genetic or it can develop due to excessive intake of dietary carbohydrates. People who have insulin resistance are at high risk for developing diabetes, as their bodies are producing plenty of insulin but their cells are not using the insulin effectively.

Unfortunately, there is no easy way to measure insulin resistance. However, if you have many of the symptoms of insulin resistance, such as elevated triglycerides, low HDL cholesterol, high blood pressure, and obesity, it is likely that you are insulin resistant. Unlike blood pressure, blood glucose, or cholesterol levels, insulin resistance is a hard thing to measure.

The good news is that a study conducted by the National

Institute of Diabetes and Digestive and Kidney Diseases (NIDDK) indicated that people with insulin resistance can reduce their risk of developing diabetes by over 50 percent by decreasing their intake of carbohydrates and increasing their level of activity.

SYNDROME X

People who are insulin resistant may also be suffering from a disorder called Metabolic Syndrome, or Syndrome X. This cluster of health problems has been recognized for at least 80 years and currently affects approximately 47 million Americans. People with Metabolic Syndrome do not necessarily have a defective metabolism, but they do have an abundance of abdominal fat, high blood pressure, poor cholesterol readings, high blood sugar, and high triglycerides. They are also insulin resistant and obese. In many cases, metabolic syndrome may be controlled by making healthier diet and exercise choices.

Sadly, many people are not making the appropriate lifestyle choices and are finding themselves among the 17 million Americans with diabetes. In 2001, the Centers for Disease Control and Prevention (CDC) printed a report in the American Diabetes Association's journal Diabetes Care predicting that diabetes, already an epidemic in the United States, is expected to increase by over 165 percent in the next 50 years. Adult-onset (type 2) diabetes is climbing at an alarming rate in younger age groups, particularly those 30 to 39 (up over 70 percent in the last ten years) and those 40 to 49 years old (up 40 percent).[3]

A first-rate scientific study supports the warnings that eating processed grains such as white rice, pasta, bread, and cold cereals is just as bad as (if not worse than) eating a lot of sugar. In February 1997, Dr. Jorge Salmeron and Harvard colleagues published the results of a study that tracked the diets of 65,173 women, ages 40 to 65, for six years. The results of this study appeared in the *Journal of the American Medical Association* and indicated that women who ate a starchy, low-fiber diet and drank a lot of soda developed diabetes two and a half times more often than women who ate a healthier diet.[4]

PHYTATES

There's another reason I'm glad high-carbohydrate diets are now becoming passé. Grains, particularly wheat, rye, and oats, unless they are sprouted, contain phytic acid, a phosphoruslike compound that interferes with calcium absorption. Phytic acid is primarily found in the husk of the grain, so there are high levels in bran. Many unsuspecting health-conscious people are washing away their calcium with daily doses of wheat or oat bran. Phytic acid also affects iron, magnesium, and zinc absorption. Mineral malabsorption is rampant these days, as evidenced by the rise in osteoporosis and increase in bone spurs, all signs of inadequate calcium metabolism.

The popularity of commercial breads may also be contributing to mineral problems. The cultivated yeast used in commercially produced breads does not remove the phytic acid from dough the way natural leavening, or sourdough, can. The natural fermentation process (in breads such as those from French Meadow Bakery) produces an enzyme that neutralizes the phytic acid. Furthermore, the longer natural leavening process breaks down the outer husks of the grain to release naturally contained minerals into the dough for greater availability to the body.

(An added advantage to naturally leavened, or sourdough, bread is its sweet taste and moist texture, kept fresh longer by a crisp crust.)

WHAT THIS BOOK OFFERS

The Super Nutrition for Women Program includes essential and healthy oils from food sources such as omega-3 rich fish and from oils such as flaxseed, sesame, olive, or macadamia. It avoids the hydrogenated fats from overly processed vegetable oils, margarine, and shortening that have been associated with disease and the problems of aging.

I emphasize variety, ensuring consumption of a wide range of vegetables, fruits, protein, low-fat and full-fat milk products, and complex carbohydrates. This means putting lean meat and eggs back into your diet; it means using all the available sources of calcium, like green leafy vegetables, not just dairy products. Variety will give your body maximum exposure to all the essential nutrients from food sources without risking the problems of excesses—gluten intolerance, yeast infections, and degenerative diseases.

With the recommended food plan, you get the fiber you need without the gluten you don't need. Rice, fruit, vegetables, and beans offer high-fiber alternatives.

You will learn not only what to include but also what to avoid. My program makes a quantum leap from the dietary model of recent decades to nutrition for the 21st century with essential fatty acids, a cornerstone for health, beauty, and immunity.

CHAPTER FOUR

Why Women Need Meat and Eggs

The human organism needs an ample supply of good building material to repair the effects of daily wear and tear.

—INDRA DEVI, YOGA TEACHER AND WRITER

The egg—a natural, egg-ceptional food! Within its shell, it has every vitamin except C; it is the best dietary source of the sulfur-bearing amino acid L-cysteine, so essential for healthy nails and skin and lustrous hair. It is an important source of trace minerals such as selenium. Its protein comes closest to matching the protein pattern best used by the body (so more of its protein's amino acids are put to use).

So why are all the beauty-conscious women who come to see me still avoiding eggs? Why are so many women choosing bran muffins or processed cereals over omelets for breakfast? Why did the USDA find that egg consumption by women dropped 37 percent between 1970 and 1995? And what are the consequences of these choices for women like Susan, the chronic dieter; Pat, the nutrition buff; and Maryann, the grabber, described in Chapter One, all of whom seldom eat eggs?

There is a disturbing trend among women who are choosing not to eat meat, especially beef. Many women proudly assert that they don't eat any red meat at all. On the other hand, their diet histories reveal plenty of cheeses, cheese spreads, gourmet ice cream, and fast-food fish sandwiches—all higher sources of dietary fat than the red meat they avoid.

Although average consumption of poultry has nearly doubled in the past twenty years, beef consumption among women has dropped over 15 percent. Can we afford to give up such an excellent source of iron, vitamins B_2 (riboflavin), B_{12}, and niacin, and zinc? Our cold, tired bodies may be giving us the answer.

What appears to be the major factor in these dietary changes is the 45-year-long crusade against cholesterol, a crusade that many experts now believe is based on faulty logic and misunderstandings about cholesterol in the diet versus cholesterol in the bloodstream.

THE BASICS OF CHOLESTEROL: HOW IT WORKS

I know you may have heard this before, but it bears repeating. Cholesterol is a waxy, fatlike substance found in foods of animal origin, such as beef, poultry, and eggs. To make sure you are adequately supplied, your liver and brain manufacture about 80 percent of the cholesterol found in your body.

Cholesterol is essential to good health. It is considered so vital that it is contained in practically every cell of the body and aids in cell membrane repair. Cholesterol in the skin reacts to sunshine to produce vitamin D. Much of the brain is composed of cholesterol, and it helps form the insulation around nerve fibers. Cholesterol is necessary for the production of cortisol, an adrenal hormone in particular demand during physical stress.

Deficiencies of cholesterol have been associated with anemia, acute infection, and excess thyroid function. Significantly
depressed cholesterol values have been found in patients with
autoimmune disorders.

Cholesterol is not soluble in water, so to travel through the
bloodstream, it is wrapped in water-soluble lipoproteins
(lipids [fats and oils] + proteins). These lipoproteins are cate-
gorized according to their protein content, or density. High-
density lipoproteins (HDLs) carry excess cholesterol to the
liver, where it is broken down to bile acids and eventually
flushed out of the body. For this reason, HDLs are referred to
as "good" cholesterol. Low-density lipoproteins (LDLs) carry
fats and cholesterol to the cells throughout the body, including the arteries, and deposit them for use.

Women under 50 tend to have higher levels of HDL than
do men in the same age range; some experts believe this may
be one factor in the lower heart attack rate among women of
this age group. Well over a decade ago, Kenneth H. Cooper,
M.D., M.P.H., director of the Aerobics Center, Dallas, Texas,
analyzed a variety of longitudinal studies and his own research
to provide guidelines for women's cholesterol levels (measured in milligrams per deciliter, mg/dl) as follows:

CARDIOVASCULAR RISK BY CHOLESTEROL AND LIPID LEVELS

Age	Total cholesterol	LDL	HDL	Triglycerides	Total-to-HDL ratio
		Low to Moderate Risk			
20–39	157–197	90–127	> 45	58–106	1.9–3.6
40–59	186–235	110–155	> 49	73–140	2.0–4.0
60+	205–252	126–175	> 50	82–146	2.0–4.8

Age	Total cholesterol	LDL	HDL	Triglycerides	Total-to-HDL ratio
High Risk*					
20–39	198–220	128–149	< 45	107–146	3.7–4.2
40–59	236–259	156–181	< 49	141–190	4.1–4.9
60+	253–276	176–198	< 50	147–206	4.9–5.5

Source: Adapted from *Controlling Cholesterol*, by Kenneth H. Cooper (New York: Bantam Books, 1988), p. 53.

* Insufficient data to definitely say that HDLs in women in this range clearly mean a high risk; this is the best estimate of risk at this time.

> = more than; < = less than.

The evidence for the belief that high levels of dietary cholesterol raise blood cholesterol levels is not as overwhelming as some would have us believe. Studies from the University of California at Los Angeles, the University of Missouri, and others find no correlation between cholesterol in the diet and heart attack rates. In a year-long Canadian study of both the Pritikin low-fat diet and the American Heart Association limited-fat diet, neither diet lowered blood cholesterol levels in patients with early vascular disease.

The present concern over cholesterol in the diet began with a Russian study in 1913 by a physiologist, Nikolai Anitschkov. He fed rabbits huge doses of cholesterol, and the cholesterol content of their blood rose dramatically by several hundred percent. This stress caused atherosclerosis, and cholesterol was found at the site of arterial damage.

Later research found that feeding rabbits pure, fresh cholesterol does not damage their arteries. However, if the cholesterol is exposed to oxygen prior to feeding, its unstable molecules produce toxic by-products. As Alan R. Gaby, M.D., a Maryland-based practitioner and nutrition author, has pointed out,

"Blood vessel damage can be produced by feeding animals even tiny amounts of these oxidation products.... Dietary cholesterol is apparently dangerous only to the extent that it becomes oxidized."[1]

According to a classic, groundbreaking study by Dr. C. B. Taylor reported in the *American Journal of Clinical Nutrition*, oxidized cholesterol from food sources that are left out at room temperature or that are fried, smoked, cured (sausage), or aged (cheese) can be highly atherogenic (plaque-producing).[2] It is not pure cholesterol that creates artery-clogging plaque, but rather the toxic substances produced by the oxidation of cholesterol. Oxidized derivatives of cholesterol are unstable and decompose into free radicals, which damage blood vessel walls.

Any animal food that has been exposed to the ravages of oxygen for extended periods of time is likely to contain chemically altered cholesterol. Cooking eggs is a good example. Hard-boiled or fried eggs produce the highest serum cholesterol; scrambled or baked eggs produce less; soft-boiled produce the least.

(Balanced with the concern for cholesterol in cooked eggs is consideration of the flulike illness caused by the bacteria *Salmonella enteritidis*, which has increased in incidence in recent years. Both the Food and Drug Administration and the USDA have found the risk of contracting the illness to be extremely small, except in some high-risk groups: the elderly, the very young, pregnant women, and people with weakened immune systems or other serious illness. To lessen the risk for these high-risk groups, the government suggests throwing out any cracked raw eggs; avoiding uncooked dishes made with raw eggs, like Caesar salad and steak tartare; cooking eggs thoroughly until both white and yolk are firm, which is likely to increase the level of cholesterol in the yolk; and storing eggs and egg dishes in the refrigerator.)

Many experts cite the Framingham study of thousands of individuals over a 14-year period as evidence in support of a low-cholesterol diet. Yet the study's director, William Kannel, M.D., has pointed out that there was "no discernable association between the amount of cholesterol in the diet and the level of cholesterol in the blood." Half the people who died of heart attacks in the study did not have high cholesterol levels.[3]

BEYOND CHOLESTEROL

Research has shown that there are better indicators of heart disease than cholesterol levels. One such indicator is homocysteine, an amino acid–type substance found in the blood. Too much homocysteine is related to a higher risk of coronary heart disease, stroke, and peripheral vascular disease. Recent studies have provided evidence of this, including a Norwegian study that followed 587 patients with coronary heart disease. Researchers found that the patients' risk of death after four to five years was proportional to their total plasma homocysteine levels. The risk rose from 3.8 percent in those with the lowest levels (below 9 micromoles [µmol] per liter) to 24.7 percent with the highest levels (greater than 15 µmol per liter).

A second indicator of heart disease involves elevated levels of C-reactive protein (CRP), a substance secreted by the liver in response to inflammatory events throughout the body. In fact, a recent finding by Dr. Paul Ridker shows that CRP levels are actually superior to LDL cholesterol in predicting cardiovascular events. Moreover, the two factors seem to be unrelated, meaning there may be a whole new way to control the risk of heart disease.

The Ridker study followed 28,000 apparently healthy women for eight years, monitoring them for myocardial infarction, ischemic stroke, coronary revascularization, or death from cardiovascular causes. The women's CRP and LDL cholesterol levels were measured at the start of the study, and factors such as age, smoking status, diabetes mellitus, blood pressure, and hormone replacement therapy were taken into account. The women who were among the top 20 percent in CRP levels were 2.3 times more likely than those in the bottom 20 percent to experience coronary heart disease. Comparatively, the women who were among the top 20 percent in LDL cholesterol had only 1.5 times the risk of their bottom 20 percent counterparts. Identifying CRP as such an important predictor of cardiovascular events may serve to explain why as many as half of all heart attacks occur in individuals with normal cholesterol levels.[4]

The good news is that the Food and Nutrition Board of the National Research Council takes the position that normal Americans will not reduce the risk of heart attack by going on a low-fat, low-cholesterol diet. Others would agree, including John Story, M.D., Purdue University; George Mann, M.D., Vanderbilt University; and Michael Oliver, president of the British Cardiac Society. Edward Ahrens, M.D., longtime cholesterol researcher at Rockefeller University, sums up the case well—to deny everyone red meat, eggs, and dairy products when only a minute fraction of the population has a problem with high cholesterol reduces the joy of life unnecessarily. And, I would add, subjects women to unnecessary nutritional deficiencies.

DIETARY ELEMENTS THAT DO
INFLUENCE HEART DISEASE

If dietary cholesterol is not the factor advertisers would have us believe, what is? Actually, not one but several factors appear particularly influential.

It is interesting to note that within the past 100 years, there has been a 350 percent increase in cardiovascular disease, but the cholesterol content of the American diet has remained about the same. Both sugar and processed oil consumption, however, have risen considerably—for example, we have increased the amount of sugar in our diet by over 30 percent since 1983.[5]

According to John Lakosa, M.D., cardiologist and chairman of the American Heart Association nutrition committee, "Saturated fats are four times more likely to raise blood cholesterol levels than dietary cholesterol itself." The liver makes cholesterol from the saturated fats, whether or not you've consumed dietary cholesterol.

Sugar also appears to play a key role in both cholesterol and triglyceride levels. Triglycerides are the substances that fill fat cells and are thought by many to be even more important than cholesterol in heart disease. Triglycerides increase in your bloodstream when you eat excessive amounts of carbohydrates from sugars in refined products, such as white flour and white sugar, fruits and fruit juices, and alcohols.

Tests at Brookhaven National Laboratory found that patients on a high-sugar, low-fat diet had triglyceride levels two to five times greater than those on a low-sugar, high-fat diet. Ancel Keys, M.D., and coworkers found that when men ate simple sugars, their serum cholesterol levels were high. These levels went down when complex carbohydrates from fruits and vegetables replaced the simple sugars (see Chapter Five for more on sugar).[6]

On the other hand, vitamin C has been shown in animals to lower blood cholesterol levels. Studies by Constance Spittle Leslie, M.D., of Pinderfields Hospital, England, have convinced her that atherosclerosis is a deficiency disease. She found that vitamin C removed cholesterol from the arteries of patients with atherosclerosis.

Animals studies have also shown vitamin B_6 deficiency to be associated with atherosclerosis. Monkeys given B_6 had their cholesterol levels lowered, even when they consumed high-cholesterol diets. When they were made deficient in B_6, they rapidly developed atherosclerosis.

Also associated with the risk of heart attack are smoking, obesity, and lack of exercise.

SHOPPING SMART

By shopping selectively, you can enjoy red meat without adding dangerous levels of saturated fats. Grass-fed or pasture-grazed beef is lower in total fat than grain-fed beef, with the added benefit of no hormones or antibiotics (see the staples shopping list in Chapter Ten for more information).

Meats are graded for quality as determined by the USDA, although there is no law requiring that packaged meats carry a label with their grade. Grading reflects appearance, flavor, and tenderness, and appears on about 75 percent of fresh beef.

The three basic grades are prime, choice, and select. Select has the lowest fat content, prime the highest. Select will usually be the least expensive, prime the most expensive. Select cuts will give you the nutrients you want without the fats that you don't want. Look especially for eye or tip of the round (with 29 percent of its calories from fat) or flank steak (34 percent) versus T-bone steak (41 percent).

MEAT, EGGS, AND MINERALS

Only about 10 percent of the population has a problem with metabolizing cholesterol. For the majority of women, avoiding red meat and eggs carries its own set of nutritional hazards.

I fully agree with Annette Natow, Ph.D., R.D., professor of nutrition at Adelphi University, New York, who was quoted in Prevention magazine, "It's almost impossible for most women to get anywhere near the iron they need from their diets."[7] The recommended daily average for premenopausal women and adolescent girls is 15 milligrams, yet the average American diet yields 6 milligrams or less for every 1,000 calories consumed. Furthermore, the body absorbs only about 10 percent of the iron consumed. Paul Saltman, a biology professor at the University of California, San Diego, estimates that 30 to 35 percent of American women have low body stores of iron.

Beef contains two and one-half times the iron of chicken. This iron, known as heme iron, is three to five times more easily absorbed than the non-heme iron of vegetables. The iron from dark green leafy vegetables is less than 10 percent absorbed, and that from brewer's yeast is less than 5 percent absorbed, while the iron in red meats is 30 percent absorbed. In addition, eating meat with iron-rich vegetables increases the absorption of the vegetable iron.

MAJOR SOURCES OF IRON

Food	Milligrams/serving
Meat, Poultry, Fish (3½ oz)	
Beef liver	8.8
Clams	6.1
Beef, lean	3.7
Shrimp	2.6
Lamb, lean	1.9
Poultry	1.5
Salmon	1.2
Beans and Lentils (1 cup)	
Limas, dry, cooked	5.6
Green split peas, cooked	4.2
Lentils, cooked	2.1
Vegetables (1 cup)	
Spinach, cooked	4.7
Peas, green, cooked	4.2
Beans, green, cooked	2.9
Fruits (1 cup)	
Prune juice	10.5
Raisins	5.6
Dates	5.3
Apricots, dried	5.1
Other	
Almonds (1 cup)	6.7
Brewer's yeast (1 oz)	4.6
Blackstrap molasses (1 tbsp)	3.2

Source: Nutritive Value of Foods (HG 72, U.S. Department of Agriculture).

Iron enables the body to maintain high energy levels by increasing the blood's oxygen-carrying capacity. It combines with protein and copper to make hemoglobin, which is the body's oxygen carrier. Tiredness and fatigue are the common signs of iron deficiency. Symptoms may come on slowly as the body depletes its stores of iron to make hemoglobin. These symptoms include weakness, headaches, tingling sensations in the hands and feet, exercise intolerance, sexual disinterest, irritability, depression, swelling of the tongue, pale lips and skin, lackluster hair, hair loss and hair thinning, and brittle nails.

Efficient muscle function depends on sufficient iron reserves, as does a good mental attitude. Iron boosts the body's resistance to stress and disease, and helps ward off invading bacteria, viruses, and infections.

USDA researchers have found that women deficient in iron have an impaired ability to maintain body temperature in the cold. Other USDA studies found that women who consumed well below the DRI (dietary reference intake) of iron woke up more frequently during the night than when their iron consumption was adequate.

Women who exercise to lose weight have an additional problem. Without adequate iron, these women's bodies burn mainly carbohydrates, not fat, for fuel during exercise. Less oxygen is used that way, but so is less fat!

Heavy menstrual flow can result in further loss of iron. This cause of iron loss can often go undetected as women become used to their menstrual cycles. Signs of excessive iron loss are most prevalent in women whose periods last longer than five days, who need to wear double pads, or who pass large clots.

Pregnancy puts such stress on the body's iron reserves that most experts agree that even a balanced diet cannot provide adequate levels of iron, so daily supplements of 30–60 milligrams are regularly prescribed. Lactating women's needs are not considered to be more than those of other women; however, supplements are usually prescribed for two to three months following birth to restore the body's iron stores.

Even women who eat red meat may not be getting full benefit from the iron they consume. The level of iron actually absorbed by the body is affected by several substances:

- Oxalic acid in fruits such as raspberries and Concord grapes, in vegetables such as dandelion greens, rhubarb, sorrel, and spinach, and in chocolate and cocoa inhibits absorption of the iron from these sources.

- Phytic acid in cereal grains and in commercial breads impedes iron as well as calcium absorption.

- Tannic acid in tea (regular and peppermint) binds with iron and prevents it from entering the bloodstream. Drinking tea with your meals can decrease iron absorption by 50 percent. If you must drink tea, have it at least one hour before or after an iron-rich meal.

- The phosphates and carbonates in soft drinks inhibit iron absorption, as do the polyphenols in coffee.

- EDTA, a widely used food preservative, can reduce iron absorption by 50 percent.

- Calcium inhibits iron absorption as well. So leave at least two hours between the time you take supplements rich in these nutrients and eating.

You can enhance your iron absorption further by eating foods high in vitamin C (tomatoes, potatoes, green peppers, dark green vegetables, citrus fruit, strawberries) just before or with your iron-rich foods. Cooking in iron pots, especially foods like tomatoes, can put additional iron into

Meat and eggs are among the best sources of vitamin B_{12} (cobalamin), another element necessary to avoid anemia. Women are urged to get 6 micrograms a day. Other sources of this valuable element are brewer's yeast, milk, sardines, mackerel, oysters, beef liver, and clams.

(Although meat and eggs do not supply folic acid, this element is also needed to prevent anemia and to assure the full use of vitamin B_{12}. It can be found in spinach, broccoli, asparagus, wheat germ, liver, orange juice, dried beans, and brewer's yeast. The DRI for women of childbearing age is 400 micrograms.)

Pork and beef are also excellent sources of zinc, another mineral commonly deficient in a woman's diet. In fact, beef has three times the zinc of chicken.

Approximately 100 enzymes in a woman's body have zinc as one of their components. Zinc is essential for the synthesis of body protein, vitamin A metabolism, proper growth, healing of wounds and burns, and development of the sex organs. It promotes the removal of harmful carbon dioxide and is directly involved in the body's metabolism of carbohydrates and energy. It forms part of the insulin component secreted by the pancreas. Zinc helps to enhance digestion, protects the body in stressful conditions, and plays an important role in many major metabolic reactions.

Zinc deficiency has been associated with lowered immunity, decreased fertility, undeveloped sex organs, poor senses of taste and smell, stretch marks, and white spots on the fingernails. In addition, chronic tiredness, hair loss, dandruff, and slow healing of wounds have been related to lack of zinc.

As I mentioned at the beginning of this chapter, eggs are one of the best dietary sources of sulfur and its transport amino acid, L-cysteine. This amino acid helps build collagen in the skin and helps transport oxygen in the bloodstream. It is necessary for the proper utilization of vitamin B_6. Sulfur itself is beneficial to skin and hair health, which may account for its being called the "beauty mineral." High levels can be found in keratin, a protein that is abundant in the horny layer of the skin, and in hair and nails.

Meat and eggs are important sources of the following other vitamins and minerals:

- **Phosphorus**—for healthy bones and teeth; formation of genetic material, cell membranes, and enzymes

- **Selenium**—antioxidant that prevents breakdown of body chemicals

- **Vitamin A**—aids in building and maintaining healthy hair, skin, and mucous membranes; needed for proper bone and tooth development

- **Vitamin B_1** (thiamin)—converts carbohydrates to energy for cells; essential to a healthy nervous system

- **Vitamin B_2** (riboflavin)—maintains healthy mucous membranes; releases energy from foods

- **Vitamin B_3** (niacin)—facilitates energy production

- **Biotin**—aids in making fatty acids; helpful in preventing hair loss; necessary to release energy from carbohydrates consumed

My plan includes up to 2 eggs a day, either prepared alone or as components of other dishes, and at least two servings (4 ounces each) of lean red meat per week. In Chapter Ten I have listed a variety of alternatives.

Getting the vitamins and minerals that we need every day is not as easy as it might seem, despite the bounty of our supermarkets. Transporting, storing, and various levels of processing often transform foodstuffs from nutrient-rich to nutrient-empty. A diet that totally excludes meat, eggs, or any entire food categories is a diet that means trouble for women. The plan that I outline in this book restores not only the variety and balance missing from so many women's diets but also the health and well-being for which these women search.

————— CHAPTER FIVE —————

Why Women Don't
Need Sugar

From disease I have learned much which life could
never have taught me in any other way.

—GOETHE

Thanks to the anti-fat crusades of government agencies and
other organizations, more and more Americans are concerned
about the kinds and amounts of fats in their diet.

What we have forgotten in our zeal is that too much
sugar—primarily the simple sugars like white table sugar,
fruits, and fruit juices—can also make fat and cholesterol in
the body the way excess nonessential saturated fat does. And it
affects calcium balance in the body as well.

Do we monitor our sugar intake as we do our fat consumption? The answer is a resounding no! And it may be
more difficult than you think. Sales of gourmet cookies, pre-
mium ice creams, and desserts laden with both sugar and fat
are at an all-time high. Sales of candy in the United States were
over $13 billion in 1997, up from about $10.3 billion in 1987,
according to industry analysts. Restaurants find an increasing

demand for the richest desserts on their menus. *Family Circle* magazine reports that their best-selling issues always feature some delectable-looking dessert on the cover—strawberry shortcake was a recent annual winner!

In fact, today you will probably eat 30 teaspoonfuls of sugar. Yes, even those of you who avoid desserts and no longer add sugar to your coffee will probably come close to consuming your weight in sugar each year.

That's because everything from cigarettes to french fries has sugar in it—added in processing or occurring naturally. Commercial brands like Hellmann's mayonnaise, Skippy peanut butter, Lipton Cup-a-Soup, Ritz crackers, and General Foods Cafe Vienna coffee all contain sugar!

Processors have discovered that sugar is not just for sweetening. Added to foods like catsup, it helps retain colors; added to baked goods, it works with yeast in the rising process and imparts a brown crust to breads and rolls; in soft drinks it adds body and texture; in chewing gum, pliability. Molasses and corn syrup may be added to a restaurant's hamburgers. Raw potato slices are often dipped in sugar water before being fried. Refined sugar, added to air-cured tobacco in the blending process, enhances both the flavor and the burning quality of cigarettes.

HOW SWEET IT WAS

A preference for sweet taste begins early—newborns given sweet liquids increase their rate of sucking. At one time, this preference may have had an evolutionary benefit. Gary Beauchamp, a biopsychologist at the University of Pennsylvania, concludes that the sweet tooth enabled prehistoric humans to select ripe fruits and berries to eat. We have, of course, long since gone beyond this straightforward connection between good taste and good food.

Our involvement with sweeteners is not only physical, but emotional as well. Consider some of the synonyms for *sweet* found in *Webster's Collegiate Dictionary: agreeable, fragrant, dear, wholesome, fresh, fine.* Where would personal relationships be without "sweetheart," "sweet talk," "sugar pie," or "sugar daddy"? Where would we be without the "sweet smell of success" and "sweetness and light"? Who would rather be a "sourpuss" than a "sweetie pie"?

Yet all is not sweetness and light with sugar. Longstanding problems with tooth decay have affected generations; although bacteria in the mouth metabolize a variety of sugars, the ability of sucrose to be converted by the bacteria into long, complex molecules that adhere to teeth to form plaque makes it especially troublesome.

The negative health effects of our love affair with sugar are being found in a wide range of illnesses. Of particular concern to women are the connections between sugar and candidiasis (yeast infections), premenstrual syndrome (PMS), excess weight, and osteoporosis, as discussed in later chapters.

SUGAR BASICS

Misconceptions about sugar abound. A case in point is a client of mine, a very successful career woman based in New York City, who called me one day to report that she was completely off sugar. Knowing of her strong sweet tooth, I asked her how she did it. She said she had gone to a well-stocked health food store and found ice cream made from rice, apple- and pineapple-juice-sweetened cookies, and candies made from barley malt. "I'm not eating any sugar anymore!"

She had fallen into the trap that so many of us do. She had simply substituted certain forms of sugar for others, but she was still eating sugar, albeit from so-called natural sources. What she had not realized was that sugar is sugar, and our bodies do not know the difference.

Like this client, when we say sugar, most of us mean refined white granulated sugar. However, there are at least a dozen other kinds, from a variety of sources:

- **Glucose** (dextrose)—the main blood sugar in our bodies, our number one energy source; present in many fruits and in the starches of vegetables such as corn.

- **Fructose**—fruit sugar from fruits, juices, and honey; commercial varieties now use corn as a base. It is twice as sweet as sucrose when added commercially to cold products and about the same sweetness as sucrose in baked goods. Because it is absorbed more slowly than sucrose, it does not raise the blood sugar level as dramatically, so it is a better sugar source for controlled diabetics.

- **Sucrose**—made up of equal portions of glucose and fructose, this is the most abundant sugar in plants; refined, usually from sugar cane or beets, it has no nutrients. It is best known as table sugar.

- **Maltose**—malt sugar, formed by the breakdown of starch.

- **Lactose**—milk sugar; less sweet than sucrose.

- **Raw sugar**—partially refined sucrose (dirt and plant debris remain, along with some trace minerals).

- **Brown sugar**—table sugar with a molasses coating.

- **Powdered sugar**—table sugar ground into fine crystals with a small amount of starch added to avoid caking.

- **Molasses**—residue after crystals of sugar are removed from beet juice or sugar cane; contains a variety of sugars. Blackstrap molasses contains measurable amounts of trace minerals, including calcium and iron.

- **Maple sugar**—sucrose made from boiling maple sap.

- **Honey**—natural syrup made up of fructose, glucose, maltose, and sucrose; sweeter than sucrose, it can raise blood sugar levels higher than sucrose does. Its composition, quality, and taste vary, with clover honey generally having more iron than other varieties.

- **Corn syrup**—derived from corn starch; made up of glucose and maltose.

- **High-fructose corn syrup**—also made from corn starch, with the fructose content increased by enzymes; sweeter than sucrose. It is now used in almost all regular soft drinks.

- **Sorbitol, mannitol, and xylitol**—synthetic products, sugar alcohols; all are more slowly absorbed than glucose and cause lower insulin responses than either glucose or sucrose. All three have laxative effects on sensitive individuals, however, and cannot be used in great quantity. When sorbitol is used to replace sugars in food products, the end result may contain even more calories because of the use of added fat needed to make the sorbitol more soluble.

These sugars share a number of characteristics:

1. They all provide four calories per gram.

2. Except for molasses, and maple syrup and honey to a lesser degree, they have no nutritional value. Whatever vitamins, minerals, and fiber that might have been present in the natural state have been removed in processing.

    Blackstrap molasses provides 14 percent of the DRI of calcium and 28 percent of iron in 1 tablespoon. Molasses, honey, and maple syrup help keep food fresher longer, so they work well as a refined sugar substitute in many recipes.

3. The negative effects seem to be the same no matter which sugar you consume.

Sugars are simple carbohydrates and are found in fruits, fruit juices, and sweeteners like white table sugar, molasses, honey, and maple syrup. Complex carbohydrates, which are chains of sugars plus protein, fats, vitamins, and minerals, are the preferred fuel for body energy. They are found in whole grains, vegetables, and beans. When complex carbohydrates are eaten, they are broken down into their simple sugars over a sustained period of time. This provides fuel and a steady release of energy.

When simple sugars and highly processed carbohydrates are eaten, they are broken down almost immediately—acting as an almost pure chemical. This rapidly releases sugar directly into the bloodstream, signaling various hormones and the pituitary gland to tell the pancreas to produce insulin. This rapid rise in the blood sugar level causes the pancreas to overreact—so much insulin is produced that the blood sugar level drops precipitously. The result is a quick burst of energy, followed by an equally fast fall in energy levels—what I call the peaks and valleys of energy. Constant stress on the clusters of special pancreatic cells, called the islets of Langerhans, to produce insulin after repeated consumption of sugary/processed foods causes these cells to become exhausted. When they no longer can produce adequate insulin levels, the result is the diagnosis of diabetes mellitus (*mellitus* comes from the Latin word for honey), commonly called diabetes.

According to a scientific study, there is one simple sugar that does *not* cause a rapid blood sugar or insulin rise. That is fructose, which provides a slower, steadier supply of blood sugar, making it the sweetener of choice for diabetics. Of all the sweetener sources that have been investigated, fructose has the slowest blood sugar rise.

In an attempt to provide a means of comparison of the effect of various foods on blood sugar levels, scientists at the University of Toronto developed the Glycemic Index. Applied to carbohydrates, including sugars, the Index helps diabetics and others interested in controlling their blood sugar levels and weight to plan their meals more effectively. In a seminal report in *Diabetes Care*, David Perkins and his associates concluded that, when included in the diet, starchy foods with a relatively low score on the Glycemic Index were associated with reductions in LDL ("bad" cholesterol) and triglyceride levels. Some of the food items in this category include legumes; pasta; grains such as barley, parboiled rice, and bulgur; and whole-grain breads such as pumpernickel. Comparing several sugars, the researchers found the average glycemic response level for maltose to be five times greater and glucose four times greater than that of fructose.

In the process of being metabolized, refined sugars rob the body of valuable nutrients—chromium, manganese, cobalt, zinc, copper, and magnesium. These nutrients are taken from the body's mineral reserves, contributing to common deficiencies in men and women.

Another factor in the deficiencies is simply the numbers—Michael Jacobson of the Center for Science in the Public Interest has summarized this point: "When you consume 20 percent of your calories from sugar, that means you have to get all of your nutrients from 80 percent of your food. It's unlikely that you're going to get them."

SWEET FAKES

Artificial sweeteners unfortunately pose their own problems. Both saccharin, a petroleum derivative, and aspartame, a combination of two naturally occurring amino acids, are referred to as "nonnutritive sweeteners," which means that they provide no calories. There are health risks associated with each of these artificial sweeteners.

A National Cancer Institute study found that certain people, primarily heavy artificial sweetener users, heavy users who smoke, and women who consume sugar substitutes or diet beverages at least twice a day, are at greater risk from the ill effects of these sweeteners than other groups.

Saccharin has been around since 1900, but its widespread use began in the late 1960s as a replacement for the banned cyclamates then in use as an artificial sweetener. In 1977 a Canadian study indicated that when pregnant rats were fed large doses of saccharin, their male offspring developed bladder cancer. As a result, the Canadians banned saccharin and the U.S. Congress ordered warning labels on all saccharin products, like Sweet 'N Low. The National Academy of Sciences in 1978 evaluated the evidence and concluded that saccharin was primarily a promoter of other cancer-causing agents, a cocarcinogen.

In the meantime, G. D. Searle developed aspartame, a combination of two amino acids and methanol (wood alcohol). Closer to sugar in taste—actually 180 to 220 times sweeter than sugar—but without the aftertaste of saccharin, aspartame was an immediate success, replacing saccharin in diet soft drinks and other food items.

Research continues on the effects of aspartame. Reports to the Food and Drug Administration and the Centers for Disease Control indicate that, as more people consume the substitute in large quantities, health may be affected. In some circumstances, individuals may be getting high levels of methanol; for example, it is estimated that on a hot day after exercise, an individual drinking three 12-ounce cans of diet cola could easily consume as much as eight times the Environmental Protection Agency's recommended limit for methanol consumption. The most common complaints are dizziness, disorientation, tunnel vision, ear buzzing, loss of equilibrium, numbing of hands and feet, inflammation of the pancreas, high blood pressure, eye hemorrhages, and seizures.

There is a newer artificial sweetener, sucralose, which has been sold under the name Splenda since 1998. It contains no calories and is intensely sweet—about 600 times sweeter than sugar. I do not recommend the use of this sweetener for a number of reasons. Sucralose is produced by chlorinating sugar to chemically change the structure of the sugar molecules by substituting three chlorine atoms for three hydroxyl groups. In my opinion, this is cause for concern, as chlorine can mimic or interfere with natural hormones like estrogen.

Few human studies have been published on the safety of

sucralose. A small study of diabetic patients using the sweetener showed a statistically significant increase in glycosylated hemoglobin (Hb A1c), which is a marker of long-term blood glucose levels and is used to assess glycemic control in diabetic patients. According to the FDA, "increases in glycosolation in hemoglobin imply lessening of control of diabetes." In all, fewer than 20 studies—none of them long-term—have been done to determine the safety of this sweetener. In terms of safety, we need to consider more than just the original substance. As the FDA notes, "Because sucralose may hydrolyze in some food products . . . the resulting hydrolysis products may also be ingested by the consumer."[1]

On average, Americans consume over 20 pounds of artificial sweetener per person per year. Artificial sweeteners can stimulate hunger or cause addictive allergies, just as sugar does. In other words, along with many of the disadvantages of sugar, we get a whole slew of proven or suspected disorders from artificial sweeteners.

SUGAR AND EXCESS WEIGHT

A four-ounce candy bar is equivalent in calories to eight average apples. Yet anyone who eats both the candy bar and the apples can tell you: the candy will not satisfy your appetite the way the apples will.

Sugar foods tend to pack a lot of calories into small packages, so you tend to eat more to feel full. Sugar also stimulates your appetite and, in many people, creates cravings.

Sugar, like damaged fats, is a dangerous source of excess calories. Absorbed quickly, unused sugar is carried to the cells, where it is converted to saturated fats (the nonessential fatty acids) and cholesterol.

These non-EFAs compete with EFAs for an enzyme, D6D, thus interfering with production of GLA and prostaglandins. As I have described, GLA activates the body's special fat-burning tissue (brown fat), which burns excess calories for heat.

Japanese researchers have found that eating fat and sugar at the same time can be more fattening than eating equivalent amounts at least an hour apart. High-fat, high-sugar foods— chocolates, French pastries, or cream pies, for example— cause you to store fat more readily. Thus, chronic dieters like Susan, who reward themselves for being careful all day by eating high-fat, high-sugar gourmet ice cream, are sabotaging their efforts at weight loss.

ARE YOU A SUGAR ADDICT?

In her continually popular book *Lick the Sugar Habit*, my friend Nancy Appleton says about herself, "I was a sugarholic." After 40 years of doughnuts, ice cream sundaes, and candy, Nancy was facing her fifth bout of pneumonia; she regularly suffered headaches, canker sores, varicose veins, and a chronic cough. She cured herself by changing her lifestyle, including eliminating sugar and chocolate from her diet.

Nancy offers a short questionnaire to analyze your own level of sugar addiction. I've reprinted it below. Answering these questions about your eating habits honestly may help you better evaluate the role of sugar in your present diet, so you can determine what, if any, changes are needed to restore your good health.

A SUGAR QUESTIONNAIRE

	True	False

1. I don't eat refined sugar every day. _____ _____

2. I can go for more than a day without eating some type of sugar-containing food. _____ _____

3. I never have cravings for sugar, coffee, chocolate, peanut butter, or alcohol. _____ _____

4. I've never hidden candy or other sweets in my home in order to find and eat them later. _____ _____

5. I can stop after one piece of candy or one bite of pastry. _____ _____

6. There are times when I have no sugar of any kind in my home. _____ _____

7. I can go for three or more hours without eating and not experience the shakes, fatigue, perspiration, irritability, depression, or anxiety. _____ _____

8. I can have candy and other sweets in my home and not eat them. _____ _____

9. I don't eat something sweet after every meal. _____ _____

10. I rarely drink coffee and eat doughnuts or sweet rolls for breakfast. _____ _____

	True	False

11. I can go for more than an hour
after waking up in the morning
without eating.　　　　　　　　　　____　　____

12. I can go from one day to the next
without drinking a soft drink.　　____　　____

Source: From *Lick the Sugar Habit* by Nancy Appleton, Ph.D. (Garden City Park, NY: Avery, 1996).

Scoring: If you marked "False" more than four times, you are probably sugar-sensitive: allergic and addicted to it. If you checked four or fewer "False" answers, you may indeed have sugar under control in your life. Or you may be fooled by the processors, unaware of just how pervasive sugar is in our diets.

BREAKING THE SUGAR HABIT

The sad fact is that even those of us who consider ourselves nutritionally aware are probably getting far more sugar than we need or want. From postage stamps to paper cups to bran flakes to hamburger buns, sugar is part of the processing. We choose fruit juice over sodas, getting more nutrients but almost the same amount of sugar. We buy sugar-free gum, unaware that the sugar alcohols used to sweeten them contain the same calories as sugar.

Just a few of the nonfood items that contain various forms of sugar are adhesives, hair spray, lozenges, tapes, aspirin, breath sprays, ointments, talcums, and toothpaste.

It would take an entire book to list the food items that contain high levels of sugar. There are many hidden sources of sugar in natural and manufactured form. Here are just a few:

HIDDEN SUGAR

Food	Serving Size	Sugar* (tsp./serving)
Lowfat yogurt, fruit	I cup	13
Fruit drink/punch	12 ounces	12
Cranberry sauce	½ cup	11.7
Beets, pickled (Del Monte)	½ cup	9.9
Frozen yogurt	½ cup	7
Regular soda	12 ounces	6–9
Angel food cake	1/12 cake	6
Jell-O Pudding Snacks	4 ounces	6
Chocolate bar	I ounce	5
Applesauce, sweetened	½ cup	4.3
Apricots, dried	4–6 halves	4
Raisins	¼ cup	4
Chocolate fudge	1½-in. square	4
Doughnut, plain	3-in. diameter	4
Frozen yogurt, low-fat	½ cup	4
Vanilla ice milk	½ cup	3.4
Vanilla ice cream	½ cup	3.1
Brownie	2×2×¾-in.	3
Orange juice	4 ounces	2.5
Applesauce, unsweetened	½ cup	2
Nature Valley granola bars	0.8 ounce	1.5
Chewing gum	I stick	0.5

Source: The U.S. Department of Agriculture, the American Dietetic Association, and the Center for Science in the Public Interest, among others.

* Approximate level of all sugars, natural and manufactured.

Some breakfast cereals may contain over 50 percent sugar, natural or added; even those that do not add marshmallows or sugar coating can be high sugar sources. Post Raisin Bran, for example, has the equivalent of 31 percent sugar in one-half cup, while Cinnamon Crunch contains 53 percent sugar in a half-cup serving. High-fiber cereals may be merely providing sugar-coated bran. While much, if not all, of the sugar in these examples is naturally occurring from the raisins, malt, and grains, sugar is sugar when it comes to many of its health effects.

Awareness, then, becomes the number one factor in controlling your sugar habit.

• Use powdered stevia to sweeten foods when necessary. Stevia is an entirely natural plant substance that is up to 300 times sweeter than sugar. This remarkable herb, native to Paraguay, has been used as a sweetener and flavor enhancer for centuries. Research done on stevia has found it to be not only safe but also effective in normalizing blood sugar levels, preventing hypertension, treating skin disorders, and preventing tooth decay. Other studies show that it is a natural antibacterial and antiviral agent as well. Stevia has been widely used in Japan since 1970, and there have been no reports of toxicity or other side effects. The active ingredient in stevia is stevioside. Unlike artificial sweeteners, it doesn't break down with heat, so you can learn to cook with it too.

• Read the label to find out if the food you eat contains sugar. Search for any of the -ose words (glucose, dextrose, sucrose, etc.). Sugar can be listed as corn sweetener, corn syrup, or just sweetener. Ingredients on labels by law are listed with the ingredient in greatest quantity shown first, the second highest listed second, and so forth.

• Make your own muffins, puddings, gelatins, sorbets, and fruit desserts, where you can control sugar content. Generally, you can cut down the amount of sugar in a recipe by one-third to one-half without affecting taste. Use unsweetened fruit juice, molasses, maple syrup, or honey as sweeteners (see recipes in Chapter Twelve).

• Substitute unsweetened fruit juice mixed half and half with mineral water or seltzer for regular or diet soft drinks or even 100 percent fruit juice.

• Use fresh fruit as snacks or desserts, but watch that you don't go overboard. They are high in natural sugar, but do carry fiber, vitamins, and minerals as well.

• Don't use sweets as rewards—for yourself or your family. More than any other food, sweets become entangled in our psychological and emotional lives: we celebrate with a cake, we console ourselves with Häagen-Dazs. Learn your own triggers and work at breaking the habit. The food diary technique has been especially helpful for many of my clients.

For more suggestions, see Chapter Twelve.

CHAPTER SIX

Controlling Those Crazy Carbohydrates

Most illnesses which befall man arise either from bad food or from excessive eating of good food.

—ANONYMOUS

Poor Pat. Like so many, she continues to believe in the low-fat, high-complex-carbohydrate diet because she enjoys bread and pasta so much. Yet she still feels tired and bloated, and fights off vaginal yeast infections. Could these problems be related to diet? Let's review the situation.

Carbohydrates—fruits, vegetables, whole grains, and beans—are a valuable source of vitamins and minerals, including vitamins A, B, and C, phosphorus, and folic acid. They are the only sources of dietary fiber. They contain the same calories per ounce as protein and less than half the calories of fat.

However, they have been linked to several health problems in today's woman. Excess consumption of carbohydrates is associated with gluten intolerance, candidiasis (yeast infections), insulin resistance, metabolic syndrome, and diabetes. As Shirley S. Lorenzani, Ph.D., wrote, "It is no coincidence that

Candida overgrowth is the twentieth century disease and sugar is the twentieth century food."[1] By enthusiastically embracing either a high-carbohydrate diet or a junk-food diet, women have once again set themselves up for ill health and needless suffering.

CANDIDIASIS AND THE CONTEMPORARY WOMAN

What are Pat's symptoms? They include an overwhelming fatigue, headaches, sinus congestion, painful joints, and repeated urinary tract infections. She was treated with antibiotics for acne as a teenager, and her only current medication is the birth control pill. In her misguided effort to avoid all fats and oils, even the essential ones, she relies on soy sauce, vinegar, mustard, and tomato sauce for taste appeal. To conform to the recommended 80 percent carbohydrate intake, she eats whole grains, and she replaces meat with pastas. When she gets hungry, she reaches for crackers, pita bread, and muffins. She is taking good care of herself. Why doesn't she feel better? Why can't her doctors find anything wrong?

This woman could be one of the estimated 90 million Americans (or one in three) experiencing symptoms of candidiasis—chronic yeast infections caused by overgrowth of the yeast *Candida albicans*. Her repeated doses of broad-spectrum antibiotics, long-term use of the birth control pill, and a diet high in carbohydrates have created the ideal biological climate in which the candida can flourish and wreak havoc on her health.

(Speaking of climate, my own experience indicates the importance of external climatic factors in candida development. Although I have practiced throughout the nation, the majority of my candida clients came from the San Francisco Bay area. San Francisco is one of my favorite cities, but its damp, rainy climate seems to contribute to flourishing candida. One of my clients with persistent candida found her problems disappeared when she moved to the drier climate of southern California.)

Perhaps as many as three-quarters of patients with candidiasis are women, for the following reasons:

1. Women suffer regular and frequent hormonal changes and imbalances as a result of the menstrual cycle, the birth control pill, and pregnancy. Such disturbances allow yeasts to grow.

2. The structure of the vagina offers a perfect home for yeasts—dark, moist recesses.

3. The structure of the female bladder and urethra is prone to infection, which is then treated with antibiotics (known activators of yeast growth).

4. Teenage girls are especially concerned about their complexion and may seek antibiotic treatment for acne.

5. Women, in general, are more likely than men to seek treatment from a physician, for everything from throat infections to menstrual difficulties, and are therefore more likely to be treated with antibiotics.

Candida is a Jekyll and Hyde microorganism. How does this normally harmless, ever-present inhabitant of our gastrointestinal system change into the source of ill health literally from our head to our toes?

Candida is a yeast, part of the huge fungi kingdom. Molds, mushrooms, mildew, and puffballs are members of the same kingdom.

Even in good health, we carry hundreds of types of yeasts and fungi—over 300 on our skin alone. The most prolific is *Candida albicans*, which prefers the gastrointestinal tract and genital area.

Normally, all these microbes live in a balanced harmony, producing substances that keep other species in check in conjunction with various activities of the immune system.

However, when the circumstances are right, candida proliferates. As its numbers grow, the noninvasive yeast changes to a more aggressive form of fungus, which bores its rootlike structures into the gastrointestinal mucosa. This allows the fungus, its toxins, and partially digested proteins into the bloodstream—and into every part of the body.

The symptoms that develop depend on the location of the yeast overgrowth and of the concentrations of toxins. Some symptoms include:

- **Gastrointestinal:** indigestion, constipation, diarrhea, abdominal pain, gastritis, bloating, mucus in stool

- **Skin:** itching, scaliness, acne, rashes

- **Eyes:** burning, blurred or erratic vision, chronic inflammation, tearing

- **Ears:** pain, deafness, fluid in ears, recurrent infection

- **Nose and sinuses:** nasal congestion, itching

- **Mouth and throat:** white patches, dry mouth, rash, sore or bleeding gums

- **Urinary/vaginal system:** recurrent bladder infection, burning or urgent urination, white vaginal discharge cystitis, vaginal burning, menstrual cramping, irregularities in period, premenstrual anxiety, or depression

- **General:** fatigue, loss of body hair, insomnia, weight loss or gain, loss of appetite, irritability, sudden mood swings, agitation, headaches, jittery behavior

Although candidiasis was described by Hippocrates in 400 B.C., it has been the recent work of physicians and researchers such as C. Orian Truss, M.D., a Birmingham, Alabama, physician specializing in diagnosing and treating candidiasis, that has begun to shed light on the factors that permit or encourage yeast overgrowth. These factors include:

A weakened immune system. Steven S. Witkin, Ph.D., published in the journal *Infections in Medicine* results of a landmark clinical study of 50 women with recurrent candida vaginal infections. He suggested that the candida infection itself appeared to decrease the body's ability to fight off future infections.[2] In fact, repeated stresses of any kind can eventually weaken the immune system. The immune system may also be deliberately weakened by steroids and other immunosuppressive drugs. Often prescribed for life-threatening or extremely debilitating conditions, such as cancer and arthritis, these drugs nevertheless carry the side effect of allowing yeasts to flourish.

Repeated treatment with broad-spectrum antibiotics. These contribute to yeast overgrowth by killing off the friendly, competitive microorganisms along with the disease-causing ones. This imbalance affects the acidity of the intestinal tract and makes additional nutrients available for more yeasts, including the bacteria killed by the drug.

Excess sugar and carbohydrates. First, when simple sugars are consumed, blood sugar (glucose) levels rise quickly and the body produces insulin to carry this glucose to the cells. When blood sugar is too high, the defending cells of the immune system become semiparalyzed. These repeated stresses on our immunity eventually break it down and yeasts begin to overgrow.

Second, sugars, including those found in fruit and starches such as potatoes and rice, are favorite foods of yeasts. Yeast cells grow and multiply rapidly in all sugars. Thus, eating sugary foods increases the likelihood that you are consuming more yeast, as well as providing food for your internal yeast cells. In addition, if carbohydrates are not fully absorbed during digestion, excesses remain in the intestine, once again providing a fertile environment for yeast.

Birth control pills. One common side effect of the use of birth control pills is vaginal yeast infections. High levels of hormones, present in the Pill, are believed to change the mucosal membrane of the vagina. These changes encourage the ever-present yeasts to overgrow.

Metabolic factors. Some experts believe that various metabolic factors encourage yeast overgrowth. For example, since copper has fungicidal properties, a deficiency or, more commonly, biounavailability of copper prevents it from acting. Copper is biounavailable when it is present in our systems but our body cannot process and use it. A stress-induced deficiency of zinc may bring this about, as may a lack of adrenal gland hormones.

Malfunctioning of any of the endocrine glands, including the thyroid as well as the adrenal glands, is thought to be a factor in some cases, besides those related to copper deficiencies. The immune system becomes ineffective after the repeated stress of hormonal imbalance, and once again yeast flourishes.

Biotin, one of the B vitamins, has been shown to prevent the yeast from converting to a more aggressive form of fungus.

Fatty acid deficiency. Japanese researchers have found that oleic acid interferes with the yeast's conversion to fungus. This

monounsaturated fatty acid is found especially in olive, macadamia nut, high-oleic sunflower and safflower, and avocado
oils, and to a lesser degree in almond, apricot kernel, peanut,
and sesame oils.

In addition, by incorporating into the structure of the
cellular membrane, the essential fatty acids decrease the per-
meability of vital tissues and organs. EFAs prevent yeast from
spreading into the bloodstream from its normal intestinal
and/or vaginal environs. The yeast cannot pass through the
intestinal wall into the circulatory system when the mucous
membrane lining of the digestive tract is strengthened by EFAs.

Clinical studies by Dr. Truss have found significant abnor-
malities in blood levels of omega-3 and omega-6 EFAs in patients with candidiasis. He also found evidence of defects in
red blood cell outer membranes in the same patients. The red
blood cells of his candida patients did not pass through the
microscopic pores of a filter as well as did normal red blood
cells, indicating rigid outer membranes.

IS CANDIDA YOUR PROBLEM?

Candidiasis is not a disorder that can or should be self-diagnosed.
However, because *Candida albicans* is so widespread, standard laboratory tests are not always definitive. The best way for you and
your physician to diagnose it may be a combination of reviewing medical history and symptoms with a trial of therapy.

The questionnaire printed below will help you and your
physician pinpoint candida's role in your current health; it
will not give you a final yes or no answer. It was prepared for
use with adults by the late William Crook, M.D., a Jackson,

Tennessee, allergist, lecturer, and author of several books, including The Yeast Connection and Women's Health, and The Yeast Connection Cookbook.

Dr. Crook spent much of his professional career writing about and battling against yeast overgrowth. He repeatedly turned up new information about this issue, and his work continues to be supported by new scientific observations and medical reports that explain how yeast relates to PMS, psoriasis, asthma, multiple sclerosis, chronic fatigue syndrome, endometriosis, interstitial cystitis, and autism.

ARE YOUR HEALTH PROBLEMS YEAST-CONNECTED?

If your answer is yes to any question, check the box in the right-hand column. When you've completed the questionnaire, add up the points you've checked. Your score will help you determine the likelihood that your health problems are yeast-connected.

	Yes	Score
1. Have you taken repeated or prolonged courses of antibiotics?	☐	4
2. Have you been bothered by recurrent vaginal, prostate, or urinary infections?	☐	3
3. Do you feel "sick all over," yet the cause hasn't been found?	☐	2
4. Are you bothered by hormone disturbances, including PMS, menstrual irregularities, sexual dysfunction, sugar cravings, low body temperature, or fatigue?	☐	2

Yes   Score

5. Are you unusually sensitive to tobacco smoke, perfumes and colognes, and chemical odors? ☐ 2

6. Are you bothered by memory or concentration problems? Do you sometimes feel "spaced out"? ☐ 2

7. Have you taken prolonged courses of prednisone or other steroids, or have you taken the Pill for more than three years? ☐ 2

8. Do some foods disagree with you or trigger your symptoms? ☐ 1

9. Do you suffer with constipation, diarrhea, bloating, or abdominal pain? ☐ 1

10. Does your skin itch, tingle, or burn; or is it unusually dry; or are you bothered by rashes? ☐ 1

Scoring for women: If your score is 9 or more, your health problems are probably yeast-connected. If your score is 12 or more, your health problems are almost certainly yeast-connected.

Scoring for men: If your score is 7 or more, your health problems are probably yeast-connected. If your score is 10 or more, your health problems are almost certainly yeast-connected.

Used with permission from *The Yeast Connection and Women's Health* by Dr. William Crook (Professional Books, 2003)

A CANDIDA PRESCRIPTION

In her classic book *Candida: A Twentieth Century Disease,* Shirley S. Lorenzani, Ph.D., points out, "It is possible to reverse Candida overgrowth without the use of anti-yeast drugs. In most cases, however, appropriate use of anti-yeast medication gives the body the boost it needs to gain the upper hand in controlling Candida."[3]

The most commonly prescribed anti-yeast drug is nystatin. This is a relatively safe, natural product made from bacterial fermentation. The few side effects that have been reported include headaches and achiness for several days after starting therapy. While it is considered the most effective of the medications available, it may nevertheless take as long as two years to bring the yeast under control.

Whether or not you and your doctor choose an anti-yeast drug as treatment, there are a variety of nutritional guidelines to follow that have been helpful to many candida sufferers. You may need to experiment to find the right combination for you. Keep in mind that many of my suggestions that appear later in this book will keep yeasts from gaining control once you have corrected the overgrowth.

1. **Avoid foods containing yeasts, molds, and the products of fermentation,** including:
   Brewer's yeast
   Raised baked goods, such as bread, rolls, pastries, pretzels
   Fermented liquors, including wine, beer, whiskey, brandy, gin, rum, vodka, cider
   Malt-containing products, such as cereals, malted milk, candies
   Vinegar and vinegar-containing foods, such as pickles,

mayonnaise, mustard, catsup, green olives, sauerkraut,. horseradish, mincemeat

Condiments like chutney, soy sauce, spices like cinnamon and black pepper, dried herbs, herb tea

Pickled and smoked meats

Mushrooms, truffles

Cheese, sour cream, buttermilk, cottage cheese, cream cheese

Dried, candied fruits (wash regular fruits thoroughly)

Fruit juices, except freshly squeezed; canned tomatoes or tomato juice, unless homemade

Melons, especially cantaloupe

2. **Avoid vitamin supplements that are yeast-based.**

3. **Avoid chronic medications that stimulate yeast growth:** steroids, birth control pills, and broad-spectrum anti-biotics. *Note:* If such medication is essential to your health, it should be continued. Do not discontinue any of these medications without consulting your physician.

4. **Avoid excessive carbohydrates,** especially sugars and gluten-rich grains, which provide a food source for the yeast. Substitute rice, millet, buckwheat, corn, amaranth, or quinoa for the gluten-containing wheat, oats, barley, and rye.

5. **Include garlic daily.** The benefits of garlic have been known for decades. In a study reported in *Mycologia* in 1977, re-searchers concluded that garlic was markedly inhibitory of all isolates of yeast-like fungi tested.[4] In fact, it is the active component in garlic, allicin, that gives it both its odor and its fungicidal properties. Garlic supplements are available (make sure the allicin has been left in), or you can eat 2 to 4 aspirin-size pieces daily (wrapping it in food helps pre-vent garlic breath).

6. **Supplement with acidophilus.** *Lactobacillus acidophilus* is one of the friendly intestinal bacteria that compete with candida and help keep the yeast under control. Various acidophilus supplements are available. In addition, although the bacterial levels are much lower than in the supplements, plain, low-fat yogurt also adds lactobacillus to your gastrointestinal system. (Frozen yogurt appears to have little, if any, helpful bacteria left, since its processing often includes a second pasteurization.)

7. **Consider nutrient supplements.** During periods of active yeast overgrowth, certain vitamins and minerals have been found deficient. According to Leo Galland, M.D., assistant clinical professor at the University of Connecticut Health Center, yeast infections affect the way the body handles magnesium, frequently increasing its excretion. In addition, vitamin B_6 is usually deficient.[5]

Food sources for magnesium include green vegetables, nuts, and seafood. Vitamin B_6 is found in organ meats, fish, soybeans, avocados, peanuts, walnuts, bananas, and other fruits.

Biotin, one of the B vitamins, prevents the yeast from converting to its more destructive fungal form. Food sources are egg yolks, organ meats, legumes, and nuts.

Your individual supplement requirements can be determined in consultation with your physician or nutritionist.

8. **Try taheebo.** Also known as pau d'arco, this herbal tea is thought to have an antifungal effect. It has proven helpful to many candida sufferers. It is available loose or in bag form in health food stores.

Once you have the candida under control, the food plan I recommend will help it stay that way. The built-in variety of fiber and grain sources will not only protect against yeast infections, but also help prevent problems with gluten intolerance and mineral loss due to excess fiber, as I explain in the next chapter.

FRANKLY FEMALE:
VITAMIN PRODUCTS FOR WOMEN

My clients have found several remedies helpful. You may want to check with your own physician or health care professional before using any of the items.

Most of the following supplements are available by calling UNIKEY, 1-800-888-4353 or visiting www.unikeyhealth.com.

Y-C Cleanse—a clinically proven homeopathic formula for the safe and effective treatment of *Candida albicans* and related yeast infections linked to bloating, allergies, fatigue, food cravings, and more. Y-C Cleanse A and B work together with your body's natural healing power to gently yet effectively treat *Candida albicans*.

Flora Key—An intestinal flora formula that helps maintain a healthy intestinal environment, Flora Key contains acidophilus, bifidus, and fructooligosaccharides (FOS). Flora Key is an unequaled formulation of viable human intestinal bacteria with Microflora Growth Concentrate and FOS. The Microflora Growth Concentrate helps reestablish and maintain healthy bacterial growth in both the small and large intestinal tracts. FOS is a type of carbohydrate that occurs naturally in certain foods. FOS stimulates growth of helpful intestinal microorganisms and is known as a probiotic. Each teaspoon of Flora Key contains approximately 6.5 billion active organisms.

Dr. Ohhira's Probiotics 12 Plus—a blend of 12 strains of live lactic acid bacteria, 10 vitamins, 8 minerals, and 18 amino acids. The most vital element of this award-winning microbiologist's product is E. *faecalis* TH10, a strain of lactic-acid-producing bacteria developed from tempeh. University studies demonstrate that the TH10 strain may be helpful in protecting against intestinal anthrax, E. *coli*, ulcer-causing H. *pylori*, and antibiotic-resistant superbugs like *Staphylococcus aureus*.

Female Multiple (Copper Free)—an all-in-one, unique supplement designed by me to meet a woman's special needs. Safe for both pregnant and breast-feeding women (contains 800 mcg of folic acid), Female Multiple is copper free, a feature that prevents unsuspected copper overload linked to fatigue, anxiety, depression, and hair loss. It also contains twice the amount of magnesium as calcium (the ideal 2:1 ratio), which optimizes calcium absorption for strong bones and relaxed muscles. The inclusion of wild yam root and dong quai maintains balanced hormone levels for women of all ages. The plant-based enzymes ensure delivery of all the essential female vitamins, minerals, antioxidants, and phytonutrients into the system.

Woman's Oil—a unique formula that I developed with Health From The Sun with the most current female beauty and health concerns in mind. Woman's Oil contains the most balanced combination of essential fatty acids and plant nutrients to bring out your best looks, health, and hormonal balance. This special blend includes EFAs from organic flaxseed oil and black currant seed oil, plus rosemary and vitamin E to nourish a woman's body and mind at any age.

Oil of oregano—a completely natural substance derived from wild oregano species. The plant grows in remote mountainous regions free of pollution. The oil is extracted using a completely natural process without chemicals or solvents. Oil of oregano is such a potent germ killer that Jean Valnet, in his book *The Practice of Aromatherapy*, noted that it is capable of sterilizing sewage. Research published in the *International Journal of Food Microbiology* showed that oil of oregano is an excellent germicide capable of killing a wide variety of fungi and bacteria. According to the *Journal of Applied Nutrition*, oil of oregano is highly effective for killing candida. Researchers in Mexico found it possesses strong antiparasitic actions, especially against giardia. I recommend the liquid oil manufactured by the North American Herb & Spice Company.

CHAPTER SEVEN

More About Controlling Carbohydrates

We have become a society of gluten gluttons.
—RICHARD A. KUNIN, M.D., PSYCHIATRIST, AUTHOR

Perhaps no episode better exemplifies what can happen to nutrition buffs than the legendary 1980s rush to oat bran. In 1987, Robert Kowalski published *The 8-Week Cholesterol Cure*, in which he highlighted the value of oat bran in lowering serum cholesterol. Within a year, sales of at least one oat bran cereal rose 600 percent! New cereals appeared almost overnight. Doughnut chains added high-calorie oat bran muffins to their sugar-laden lineup.

Millions of cholesterol-fearing people eagerly embraced this single food item; they enthusiastically added various oat products, not just the bran, to their diet in the belief that if a little is good, a lot is better. Consuming oats and other grains at every meal and as snacks, however, does not lead to health: it can cause malabsorption of essential vitamins and minerals from too much fiber, and it can bring about pain, discomfort, and a lifelong intolerance of the gluten-containing grains wheat, oats, rye, and barley.

Following the publication of my first book, *Beyond Pritikin*, I received a telephone call from a Florida newspaper reporter wanting an extensive interview. He had purchased the book and after reading it had implemented my suggestions for individuals with symptoms of gluten intolerance. He had stopped eating his daily sandwiches on whole-wheat bread, and his chronic stomach pains, from which he had suffered for almost two years since beginning a high-complex-carbohydrate diet, had disappeared almost overnight. His relief over this simple change in his diet was typical of the response of my clients with similar complaints.

The most serious form of gluten intolerance is celiac disease. Dr. Allessio Fasano, a pediatric gastroenterologist at the University of Maryland, believes that celiac disease affects one in 150 individuals. However, consuming gluten-rich foods can be a problem for those of us without the celiac gene. As reported in the *Los Angeles Times* in 2002, millions of Americans suffer from abdominal bloating and fatigue after eating gluten-containing grains.[1]

THE STAFF OF LIFE?

Despite the increased interest in oats, wheat remains the overwhelming favorite in terms of use, representing more than 80 percent of our total grain consumption. As I discussed in Chapter Three, several factors have brought about a 20 percent increase in wheat consumption within a 15-year period:

expanded vegetarianism, increased interest in pastas and grain-based ethnic cuisines, and a heightened awareness of the value of fiber.

Most important, however, is the versatility of gluten from wheat and other grains in enhancing processed foods. Gluten is a naturally occurring water-soluble complex protein that gives elasticity and extensibility to grain flours and products made with them. Sophisticated food technologists continue to find new uses for gluten:

• As an adhesive in breading to coat foods

• As a stabilizer and to add body to beverages

• As a glaze over meat patties and other processed meats

• As an expander (gluten quickly absorbs about twice its weight in water)

• As a tableting aid in pharmaceuticals

Gluten is a component of modified food starch, which is used in almost all processed foods. It is needed to make monosodium glutamate (MSG) and other flavor-enhancers. Wheat flour may be hidden in ice cream, catsup, mayonnaise, and even instant coffee.

In his practice, nutrition pioneer Richard Kunin, M.D., author of *Mega-Nutrition for Women*, has noted that the majority of patients have some kind of symptom related to minor gluten malabsorption. "A one-sided preference for grains can spell trouble for many people because of a relatively common weak link in the metabolic ability to process these grains," he says.

Unable to handle this gluten overload, many of us develop symptoms of minor gluten malabsorption: fatigue, persistent intestinal gas, bloating within a couple of hours of eating, bowel irregularities, frequent diarrhea, and folic acid deficiency. Others of us develop full-scale gluten intolerance with additional symptoms of irritable bowel, weakness, a tendency to bleed, muscle cramps, bone pain, anemia, headache, and poor appetite.

No matter what the severity, gluten intolerance involves an alteration of the cellular lining of the small intestine. Gluten causes the villi of the lining to flatten. Since these fingerlike structures are responsible for absorption of nutrients, when gluten is present, proteins, fats, carbohydrates, iron, calcium, folic acid, and vitamins D and K are not properly absorbed. Major deficiencies can develop. In women, this may mean menstrual irregularities, infertility, osteoporosis, and anemia, in particular.

Untreated gluten intolerance can lead to intestinal cancer or ulceration, and neurological disorders. In fact, a number of studies are being conducted to examine further the observed associations between gluten intolerance and multiple sclerosis, autism, schizophrenia, rheumatoid arthritis, certain skin conditions, and diabetes.[2]

I first became aware of these issues through the early work of the late researcher F. Curtis Dohan, M.D. Dr. Dohan, at the Eastern Pennsylvania Psychiatric Institute, Philadelphia, spent more than 30 years investigating schizophrenia and diet. In one study, twice as many patients who were on a diet free of both cereal and milk in a high-security ward were able to return to the minimum-security ward than those who were on a high-cereal diet. As early as 1966, Dr. Dohan noted that psychoses occurred more often in gluten-intolerant individuals than was predicted by chance. In addition, he has reported that certain substances were found in the urine of both schizophrenics and celiacs.

Research from Berkeley, California, indicates that milk and wheat proteins break down into the same sequence of amino acids during digestion. This may account for the observed frequency of lactose intolerance among the gluten intolerant.

Other studies that have analyzed wheat consumption and schizophrenia incidence statistics report that places where wheat is the staple grain experience higher levels of diagnosed schizophrenia than those in which nongluten grains were staples. For example, a study of 65,000 residents of the highlands of New Guinea, where little or no grain is consumed, found only two chronic schizophrenics; in the coastal area of the same country, wheat is a staple in the diet and schizophrenia occurred about three times as often. In Indonesia, populations of adults who ate grains had a schizophrenia rate of 9.7 per 1,000 people, whereas those whose diet did not include grain had no schizophrenia cases.

In my own practice, one client, a manic-depressive, was referred to me by her psychiatrist for nutritional counseling. Her diet history revealed excessive amounts of gluten-based grains: bagels every morning, muffins as an evening snack, sandwiches as a lunchtime staple, plus, of course, a wide variety of processed foods, which often contained wheat flour. Within three weeks of starting a diet minus gluten-based products, she reported feeling better able to cope, and her mental outlook was markedly improved. She told me that she felt much less confused and "clearer" for the first time in a long time. She was able to make decisions and stick to them. After keeping a detailed diet history for two months, she was able to see for herself that when she cheated, her mental well-being was negatively affected. Keeping to a wheat-free diet was essential to her clarity of mind. This client eventually developed a food service that specialized in healthy foods.

OVERCOMING GLUTEN INTOLERANCE AND OTHER CARB-RELATED DISORDERS

You may be thinking, "I don't eat *that* much grain." However, when you monitor your food intake with a food diary, you may find more than you thought: cereal for breakfast, a muffin at midmorning, two slices of bread on a lunchtime sandwich, pasta with bread at dinner, and cookies before bed, to be repeated with variations day after day. The more processed foods you eat, the greater your intake of hidden gluten as well. It quickly adds up to much more than your system was designed to handle.

Because of the serious long-term consequences of untreated gluten intolerance, it is essential to consult your physician.

Gluten intolerance, insulin resistance, and diabetes can develop at any age. Therefore, it is important to learn what to avoid and what to include in your diet. For individuals with minor malabsorption, skipping wheat, oats, rye, and barley in products such as baked goods, pastas, and cereals may be enough to allay symptoms. Fiber is contained in a variety of complex carbohydrate sources. Vary your grain choices to avoid overload; grains like rice, millet, corn, and buckwheat are tasty, nutritional nongluten alternatives. Starchy vegetables like squash and sweet potatoes can nutritionally replace grain-based dishes, providing fiber, vitamins, and minerals.

Those with full-scale gluten intolerance should avoid a wide variety of foods.

Foods to Avoid[3]

Commercial beverages and fruit juices—ale, beer, gin, whiskey, instant coffee, cocoa, drinking chocolate, malted milk powder, Ovaltine, Postum, tomato juice

Baked goods—all commercial baked goods, including breads, cakes, cookies, crackers, doughnuts, muffins, pancakes, pastries, waffles, bagels, dinner rolls, crispbread, breadcrumbs, matzoh, pretzels, rusks; baking powder

Candy—all filled chocolates, toffees, fudge, caramel, marzipan, chewing gums

Cereals and grains—all cereals containing wheat, barley, rye, or oats; only cereals guaranteed gluten-free should be consumed (puffed rice, crisped rice, and cornflakes are generally safe); dumplings, macaroni, noodles, spaghetti, vermicelli, semolina

Dairy products—synthetic cream, malted milk, cheese spreads

Desserts and puddings—all pies, dessert mixes, custard powders, instant desserts, rennet powder or tablets, lemon pie filling, lemon/orange curds, lemon powders, trifle and other desserts with cake ingredients

Fats—commercial salad dressings, mayonnaise

Fish—pickled herring and other pickled fish, frozen breaded fish, fish packaged in sauce, fish paste

Flours—all flours containing the grains of wheat, barley, rye, and oats

Fruit—baby preparations, glacéed fruit

Gravies—gravy thickeners and mixes

Ice cream—all commercial types plus, of course, cones, wafers, crumb toppings

Meats—all commercial preparations containing fillings, such as sausages, luncheon meats, meat pies, mincemeat, frankfurters, meat pastes; canned meat

Sauces and condiments—thickened sauces, bottled sauces, pickles, anchovy sauce, catsup, horseradish sauce
Snacks—potato chips, french-fried potatoes
Soups—all canned and dried soups, all thickened soups, all creamed soups
Spices—celery salt, chutney, curry powder, mustard
Spreads—fish paste, meat spread, cheese spreads, processed peanut butter, sandwich spreads
Vegetables—vegetables in sauces, mayonnaise, or cream; baby foods; vegetable mixes

Note that some products are guaranteed gluten-free by the manufacturer. However, so many processed foods contain MSG and other hidden gluten sources that if you have any doubt at all, you should avoid the food.

While this list may seem long and may contain some standards in your diet, especially if you are a grabber like Maryann or a nutrition buff like Pat, the list of available foods is equally varied. In fact, my list of Super Foods for Super Women, with modification of the choice of grains, provides the basis for a healthful, gluten-free lifestyle.

Foods to Enjoy

Fruits—all fresh or frozen ones; juices except tomato; apple and other fruit sauces; dried fruits
Vegetables—all fresh, frozen, or canned, as long as they do not have sauces; raw or cooked, including steamed, boiled, roasted
Carbohydrates—brown rice, millet, buckwheat, corn, amaranth, quinoa; lentils, dried peas, butter beans; potatoes, parsnips, pumpkin

Proteins—meats, including lean beef, lamb, veal (except as
noted above); fish; poultry; cheese; eggs; soybeans
Fats—100 percent cold expeller-pressed natural oils

See the shopping list in Chapter Ten for more detailed information on the food staples.

A NOTE ABOUT NONGLUTEN GRAINS

While gluten-free white flour is available, it is a refined product, devoid of the vitamins, minerals, and fiber of whole grains.
Therefore, it is not a recommended substitute. I recommend
more emphasis on the gluten-free grains: rice, millet, corn,
buckwheat, and the best from the shelves of natural food stores,
such as amaranth, quinoa, teff, and spelt. Be sure to check out
Healthseed Spelt Bread from French Meadow Bakery, and the
Original Sprouted Ezekiel 4:9 Bread from Rainier. These breads
are sold in the frozen bread section, fresh bread section, and by
mail order.

Healthseed Spelt is packed with flax, pumpkin, and sunflower seeds for added crunch. Instead of yeast, the bread is
naturally leavened with fermenting agents that break down the
flour's cellulose structure, neutralize its mineral-inhibiting
phytic acid, and release more nutrients into the dough. Ezekiel
4:9 Bread is also a flourless whole-grain bread that I have recommended for years. It does have a small amount of sweeteners (either molasses or barley malt).

Flours from potatoes, soy, rice, and tapioca can successfully
be used in cooking. Gluten-intolerant individuals may find
they are intolerant to some or all of these as well, so experiment with your own diet.

Quinoa, known as the mother grain of the Inca civilization, contains one of the highest levels of protein of any grain, with an average of 16 percent compared with 14 percent in wheat, 9 percent in millet, and 7 percent in rice. The seed is rich in the amino acid lysine, so helpful in curbing herpes viruses and ridding the body of metabolized lipoproteins. It has the same amount of calcium as low-fat milk, with four times the phosphorus. It is also a good source of B vitamins and vitamin C.

This chart compares quinoa with several gluten and non-gluten grains for its nutritional and dietary fiber content, expressed in percentages.

NUTRITIONAL AND FIBER CONTENT OF SELECTED GRAINS (PERCENTAGES)

	Water	Protein	Fat	Carbohydrates	Fiber	Ash
Quinoa	11.4	16.2	6.9	63.9	3.5	3.3
Wheat	13.0	14.0	2.2	69.1	2.3	1.7
Oats	12.5	13.0	5.4	66.1	10.6	3.0
Rice	12.0	7.5	1.9	77.4	0.9	1.2
Buckwheat	11.0	11.7	2.4	72.9	9.9	2.0

Source: *Lupine and Quinoa*, by I. Junge (Chile: University of Concepcion Publication, 1973) and U.S.D.A.

After cooking, quinoa quadruples in size, yet retains its crunchiness. It can be used in salads, as a substitute for couscous, as a side dish mixed with pesto, or a stuffing for poultry or vegetables.

It is available from health food and specialty stores; it is imported by: Quinoa Corp., P.O. Box 279, Gardena, CA 90248, www.quinoa.net.

Amaranth is also a South–Central American grain high in protein, measuring some 16 to 18 percent. It is high in vitamins A, B, and C, calcium, and fiber. Amaranth flour is used in cookies, crusts, crackers, cakes, muffins, pancakes, breads, and pocket breads. Breakfast cereals are also available that feature amaranth. Please keep in mind that many gluten-sensitive people make the mistake of giving up gluten grains only to eat too many nongluten grains and sugars. This can lead to carbohydrate sensitivity, insulin resistance, metabolic syndrome, and type 2 diabetes. To prevent exchanging one health problem for another, make sure to substitute plenty of multicolored vegetables in place of gluten-filled grains.

WHAT ABOUT FIBER?

Individuals who currently rely on bran cereals for their fiber may not realize that there are many delicious, inexpensive, gluten-free fiber alternatives. And, yes, there are even alternatives to oat bran that have the same cholesterol-reducing properties.

Fiber is the indigestible part of plant foods. There are several kinds, including pectins, gums, cellulose, and mucilages. Some are insoluble because they do not dissolve in water. Insoluble fibers include the fiber contained in wheat and corn bran, grains, nuts, some vegetables, and flaxseed. Insoluble fibers absorb water as they move through the intestines, increasing the size of the stool. This helps waste materials to move out at a faster pace, a process believed to contribute to the lower rates of colon and rectal cancer among those eating high-fiber diets. The fiber is thought to reduce the time cancer-causing substances spend in the intestines and to dilute their concentration. Insoluble fiber is also helpful in bowel disorders such as constipation and diverticular disease, in which weakened areas of the intestine wall become inflamed.

However, due to its coarseness, too much insoluble fiber may irritate the bowel. Another problem with grain fiber, especially wheat bran, is that it can interfere with the absorption of crucial female minerals, including calcium, magnesium, iron, and zinc. Given the low intake of these minerals by many women, increased excretion stimulated by too much fiber can only add to the likelihood of deficiency and ill health.

Soluble fiber, which dissolves in water, is rich in pectins and gums. Oat bran, barley, black-eyed peas, fresh vegetables like carrots and okra, fresh fruits like apples, prunes, and grapefruit, and flaxseeds, are rich sources of soluble fiber.

What about oat bran's cholesterol-reducing powers? It is the soluble fiber in the oats that has been shown to lower cholesterol, in one study by 36 mg/dl, in another by 10.6 percent. However, pectin (fruit fiber), psyllium seed husks, and guar gum (a bean fiber) have all proven helpful in lowering blood cholesterol levels in clinical studies.

Other studies have found particular health benefits of soluble fiber for diabetics. For example, James W. Anderson, M.D., of the Veterans Administration Hospital, Lexington, Kentucky, studied the effects of a high-carbohydrate, high-fiber diet on diabetics. He found that when carbohydrates are eaten with fiber, the blood sugar levels did not rise as high as when carbohydrates were eaten alone, so the diabetics required less insulin. The fiber slowed the absorption of the carbohydrates.

Another study at the University of Bristol, England, found that fiber lowered the demand for insulin in healthy subjects and produced a longer-lasting feeling of fullness—news for women trying to avoid overeating. When individuals were given apple juice, the insulin level in their blood rose twice as high as that of individuals who ate an equivalent amount of whole apples. Furthermore, by the time blood sugar levels had returned to normal in the whole-apple group, the levels were clearly below normal in the juice group, a response usually associated with hunger pangs.

FIBER ALTERNATIVES

The average American diet contains about 11 grams of fiber. Recommended levels are 25 to 35 grams to optimize the cancer-prevention, cholesterol-lowering, and intestinal cleansing effects. A diet that emphasizes unrefined, unprocessed fresh foods, such as the plan described in this book, will enable you to meet these recommendations without counting grams. Here is a list of the fiber content of various high-fiber, nongluten foods, along with some suggestions for food choices that will increase your intake of dietary fiber.

HIGH-FIBER FOODS

Food	Serving Size	Grams Dietary Fiber
Acorn squash, cooked	½ cup	3.6
Almonds, chopped	2 tablespoons	2.2
Apple, with peel	1 medium	2.8
Asparagus, cooked	¾ cup	3.1
Blackberries, fresh	½ cup	4.5

Food	Serving Size	Grams Dietary Fiber
Black-eyed peas, cooked	½ cup	12.4
Broccoli, raw	½ cup	2.5
Brussels sprouts, cooked	½ cup	3.9
Carrots, cooked	½ cup	2.3
Carrots, raw	1 medium	3.7
Corn, vacuum packed	½ cup	6.0
Green beans, cooked	½ cup	2.3
Green peas, young, canned	½ cup	7.9
Kale, cooked	½ cup	2.8
Kidney beans, canned	½ cup	7.9
Lentils, cooked	½ cup	2.0
Nectarine	1 small	1.7
Onion, raw, chopped	½ cup	2.6
Pear, fresh	1 medium	5.0
Pinto beans, cooked	½ cup	5.3
Potato, white, baked with skin	1 medium	3.8
Prunes, cooked	⅓ cup	5.8
Raspberries, red, fresh	¾ cup	6.8
Sauerkraut, canned	½ cup	2.4
Spinach, canned	½ cup	2.5
Spinach, raw	2 large leaves	1.8
Split peas, cooked	½ cup	5.1
Strawberries, fresh	¾ cup	2.0
Sweet potato, cooked	1 large	4.2
Zucchini, cooked, sliced	½ cup	2.7

Source: Adapted from *Plant Fiber in Foods*, by James W. Anderson, M.D. (Lexington, KY: HCF Diabetes Research Foundation).

FIBER FIXES WITHOUT THE GLUTEN

• Eat the whole fruit rather than the juice—all the vitamins plus the fiber, with less concentrated sugar.

• High-fiber lunches include lentil, split pea, or black bean soup; vegetarian chili; a bean burrito; or a steamed vegetable plate with a topping of lightly toasted ground flaxseeds.

• At the salad bar, look for sprouts, peas, garbanzo beans, raw cauliflower, broccoli, and zucchini to add to your greens.

• A sweet potato has 4.2 grams of fiber per potato. Use it as a side dish instead of pasta. Try making sweet potato muffins or bread with nongluten flour, instead of oat bran muffins.

• Snack on raw vegetables or air-popped popcorn for a high-fiber fill-up.

• Add puréed vegetables such as beans or peas to thicken sauces or soups.

• Serve fruits and vegetables unpeeled whenever possible. Nutrients as well as fiber are often stored there.

FIBER CHOICES

Instead of	Choose
White rice	Brown rice
Apple juice	Whole raw apple
Hamburger on bun	Chili with beans
Salami on hard roll	Bean taco with lettuce/tomato
Chicken noodle soup	Lentil soup
Lettuce salad	Spinach salad

Instead of	Choose
Strawberry ice cream	Strawberries
Macaroni salad	Three-bean salad

Fiber has finally "come out of the closet" and, given the research findings about its health benefits, it deserves to stay out for good. However, to make the most of these benefits, think of fiber as an integral part of your food choices from unrefined foods and grains, rather than as a separate food additive to be tolerated by sprinkling it on other foods. Gradually replace low-fiber foods with high-fiber ones and you will establish a new eating pattern that you can maintain throughout your life without wreaking havoc on your digestive system.

CHAPTER EIGHT

What Women Miss About Calcium

The only way to keep your health is to eat what you
don't want, drink what you don't like, and do what
you'd rather not.

—MARK TWAIN

According to the Centers for Disease Control, 90 percent of
American women are calcium deficient on a daily basis. They
risk gum disease, menstrual cramping, depression, insomnia,
and, in their future, osteoporosis, the brittle bone disease. If we
briefly review the three diet styles I have referred to throughout
this book, I think you'll see why such a deficiency exists.

Susan, the chronic dieter, takes in fewer calories and, of
course, fewer nutrients than her nondieting colleagues. She
skips the calories of dairy products for the zero calories of diet
soft drinks. Should her dieting begin to affect her menstrual
cycle, she could experience disruptions in estrogen production. Low dietary intake of calcium, magnesium, and boron;
low estrogen levels; and excess phosphorus, from the soft
drinks, are all negative factors in the complex process of calcium absorption.

The nutrition buff, Pat, has her share of calcium disrupters. Embracing the high-carbohydrate, low-fat dietary model, she, too, avoids dairy products. While she gets some alternative calcium sources in her vegetables, the oxalic acid in several of them and the phytic acid in the many grains she eats work to inhibit calcium absorption.

Grabbers like Maryann tend to eat too much salt, caffeine, bad fats, and sugar. The processed foods they reach for are frequently deficient in the calcium-aiding nutrients magnesium, boron, and vitamins C, D, and K. As I will explain, all of these factors, along with several others, affect the body's ability to use what calcium is present, contributing to postmenopausal osteoporosis.

PUTTING CALCIUM TO USE: HOW IT WORKS

No matter how much calcium you take in, a certain amount will pass through the intestine and kidneys and be lost through excretion. This process protects the neuromuscular system, preventing muscle spasm. In addition, the level of calcium carried in the blood at all times must stay between 9 and 11 mg/dl. This means that if calcium intake is low, the body must get calcium from another source in order to maintain the blood calcium level.

When blood calcium levels drop, the parathyroid gland sends out a hormone that signals osteoclasts, which break down bone, to release calcium being stored in the bones. This calcium restores the level in the blood to normal.

If calcium levels are too high, another hormone stimulates production osteoblasts, which tie up the excess calcium by making new bone.

While 99 percent of our body's calcium is in our bones, the other 1 percent in our blood, fluids, and soft tissue is critical to the proper functioning of every cell. This accounts for the complex system designed to maintain these calcium levels, no matter what our dietary intake. Calcium plays a critical role in blood clotting, cell division, muscle contractions and maintenance of tone, brain function, hormonal balance, and even heartbeat. It has a sedative effect (remember Mom's glass of warm milk before bed) and serves as a nerve tranquilizer. Research at New York Hospital–Cornell Medical Center has found that calcium can lower blood pressure in certain individuals. Other studies point to a lower risk of colon cancer with adequate calcium levels.

The body cannot manufacture calcium, so the mineral must come from our diet or supplements. Symptoms of severe blood calcium deficiency include painful muscle contractions, tremors, and convulsions; lesser deficiencies may bring on heart palpitations, backaches, bone pain, insomnia, numbness, and menstrual cramps. Inflamed and bleeding gums (other than those caused by a vitamin C deficiency) are frequently an early warning sign of significant depletion of bone calcium—osteoporosis.

THE INHIBITORS

Even if you take in the recommended amount of calcium in your daily diet, certain factors can affect calcium metabolism and absorption, causing calcium deficiency. These factors include:

- A diet that is high in fat, protein, or sodium
- Imbalances in the calcium-phosphorus ratio

- Aluminum intake

- Oxalates from coca, dandelion greens, sorrel, rhubarb, and spinach

- Phytic acid and excess fiber from grains and bran

- Caffeine

- Cigarette smoking

- Inadequate hydrochloric acid in the stomach for digestion

- Certain drugs and over-the-counter medications

Excesses in Diet

A high-protein diet brings excess nitrogen and sulfur into the blood, which sets up an acid condition that leaches calcium from the bone to neutralize the condition. High levels of the wrong fats combine with calcium in the intestines, forming insoluble compounds that make the calcium unusable. Excess sodium causes calcium to be excreted in urine; this, in turn, lowers blood calcium levels, signaling the hormone system to cause calcium to be withdrawn from bones.

Calcium-Phosphorus Balance

The calcium-phosphorus ratio is a vital factor in the optimal use of calcium. About one-fourth of the mineral content of your body is phosphorus, most of it tied up as calcium phosphate. Experts believe we need approximately a 1.2:1 ratio of calcium to phosphorus (an average of 1,000 milligrams calcium to 800 milligrams phosphorus daily) to keep the calcium absorption process in balance. Too much sugar lowers

the blood phosphorus level. Excesses in phosphorus build up
in a diet high in red meat, poultry, and carbonated soft drinks.
Meats like pork chops and ham contain up to 30 times more
phosphorus than calcium. Chicken contains more phosphorus (250 milligrams in 3½ ounces) than even lean cuts of red
meat (158 milligrams in 3½ ounces of ground lean beef).

Soft drinks contain phosphoric acid, a phosphorus-
containing substance. The soda does not, however, contain an
equivalent amount of calcium to maintain the necessary
calcium-phosphorus balance. Soft drinks containing the highest levels of phosphorus include Tab, Diet Coke, Coca-Cola,
Caffeine-Free Coke, and Mr. Pibb.

Aluminum

Aluminum affects both phosphorus and calcium. According
to a seminal article published in *Gastroenterology*, small amounts
of aluminum-containing antacids, taken three or four times a
day for two to five weeks, inhibited absorption of phosphorus
and increased the excretion of calcium in urine and feces, especially in individuals with low calcium intake.[1] Taking more
than 2 teaspoons of these antacids a day can begin to affect
your calcium levels.

It is interesting to note that some antacids like Tums are
good sources of calcium. Tums contains calcium carbonate,
but no aluminum. Its use as a supplement should be moder-
ated, though, since it contains both sucrose and talc.

Aluminum is found in many antacids (Maalox, Amphojel,
Gelusil, Mylanta); in foods cooked in aluminum pans or
wrapped in foil; in beverages served in aluminum cans; in
many local drinking water supplies (fluoridation adds to
the problem by leaching aluminum into the water from the

surrounding storage areas); in pickles; in peppermint tea; and in processed cheeses, cheese spreads, and cream cheese.

Oxalates and Phytates

Some foods contain natural substances that interfere with calcium absorption. For example, spinach is high in calcium, but it contains calcium-blocking oxalates. So do cocoa, asparagus, sorrel, rhubarb, and dandelion greens. The oxalic acid they contain binds with the calcium to form calcium oxalate, which is indigestible.

Grains have phytic acid, a phosphoruslike compound which combines with calcium in the intestine and blocks its absorption. In excess (as in some vegetarian and high-carbohydrate diets), grains also provide too much insoluble fiber, which binds with the calcium and carries it out of the body, unused. Try to avoid eating foods high in oxalate and phytic acid with calcium-rich meals.

Caffeine

Caffeine, from coffee, tea, and soft drinks, doubles the rate of calcium excretion. Three cups of black coffee can result in a 45-milligram calcium loss.

Cigarette Smoking

In her book The Calcium Plus Workbook, Evelyn Whitlock, M.D., highlights the role of cigarette smoking: "Smoking doubles the risk of osteoporosis, decreases the effectiveness of estrogen, is associated with early menopause and worsens the detrimental effects of chronic underweight on the skeleton. The bad news about smoking just keeps getting worse!"[2]

In several groundbreaking studies three-quarters of the women who developed osteoporosis are or were smokers, most of whom smoked at least a pack a day. Some animal studies have shown demineralization of bone when there are high blood levels of cadmium, such as that found in the blood of cigarette smokers. Other studies point to the altered level of estrogen and other hormones brought about by cigarettes. Women who smoke a pack a day begin menopause an average of two years earlier than nonsmokers.

Hydrochloric Acid

As we age, our ability to absorb calcium declines: in women, this process begins in their 40s, in men not until their 60s. Our bodies also produce less hydrochloric acid. A study by Drs. Robert Heaney and Robert Recker of Creighton University, Omaha, found poor calcium absorption in middle-aged women who did not secrete adequate stomach acid.

Consumption of carbonated soft drinks can contribute to this problem in women of all ages. The beverages neutralize hydrochloric acid, thereby making it ineffective for digestion and calcium absorption.

Drugs and Calcium

A number of drugs have been found to interact with calcium or its enhancer, vitamin D. Some act to increase excretion, others block absorption. Here are the common ones:

CALCIUM AND VITAMIN D EFFECTS OF
COMMON PRESCRIPTION DRUGS

Drug	Calcium Effect	Vitamin D Effect
Anticonvulsants		
Dilantin	*	Decreased absorption
Phenobarbital	*	Increased inactivation
Primidone	*	Increased inactivation
Sedatives		
Glutethimide	*	Decreased absorption, increased inactivation
Antacids		
Aluminum hydroxide	Increased urinary excretion	Can cause vitamin D deficiency
Maalox or Mylanta	Decreased absorption	—
Laxatives		
Mineral oil	*	Decreased absorption
Phenolphthalein	Decreased absorption	Decreased absorption
Steroids		
	Decreased absorption, increased excretion, decreased bone formation, increased bone breakdown	Decreased activation
Diuretics		
Furosemide, ethacrynic acid, triamterene	Increased urinary excretion	—
Chlorothiazide, hydrochlorothiazide	Lowered urinary calcium	—

Drug	Calcium Effect	Vitamin D Effect
Other Substances		
Thyroid hormone	Increased urinary excretion, increased loss in sweat	—
Tetracycline	Decreased absorption	—
Vitamin A (75,000 IU)	Increased urinary loss	—
Cholestyramine	*	Decreased absorption
Para-amino salicylic acid	?	May cause vitamin D malabsorption from fat malabsorption
Methotrexate	Calcium loss	—
Sulfur-containing amino acids	Increased urinary loss	—

Source: *The Calcium Plus Workbook*, by Evelyn P. Whitlock, M.D. (New Canaan, CT: Keats Publishing, 1988). Copyright 1988 by Evelyn P. Whitlock.

* May show decreased absorption due to vitamin D effects.

THE ENHANCERS

With so many inhibitors, it is not surprising that over 25 million Americans suffer from osteoporosis brought on by inadequate calcium. However, there are several enhancers of calcium absorption, including:

• Magnesium

• Vitamins C, D, and K

• Boron and silicon (trace minerals)

- Estrogen

- Exercise

Magnesium

Magnesium acts in concert with calcium and phosphorus. It is vital for calcium metabolism and transport into bone and soft tissues; it helps prevent formation of calcium oxalate crystals (kidney stones). I suggest a ratio of one part magnesium to one part calcium for optimal bone health, and ideally a ratio of two parts magnesium to one part calcium, where the calcium comes primarily from food.

The Enhancing Vitamins

Several vitamins are valuable for adequate calcium absorption. Vitamin C is one enhancer. Vitamin D is essential for calcium to be transformed into a usable form. It increases calcium absorption in the small intestine and calcium retention by the kidneys, and it helps the action of the parathyroid hormone to release calcium from the bone. Vitamin D is made in the skin, with the help of the essential fatty acids, in the presence of sunlight. Spending one hour in the sun will produce about 600 units of vitamin D, more than the recommended daily allowance. (There are a number of drugs that interfere with vitamin D; see the chart on pages 121–122.)

Preliminary studies indicate a role for vitamin K in maintaining bone strength. A report in *The Journal of Clinical Endocrinology and Metabolism* indicates that people with osteoporosis had low levels of vitamin K. When levels were normalized, bone density increased and bone loss decreased.[3]

The Enhancing Trace Elements

As research into osteoporosis and bone fragility continues, new relationships have emerged, albeit not always clearly defined. For example, researchers at the U.S. Department of Agriculture found that boron plays a key role in maintaining calcium and magnesium levels by helping the body synthesize both estrogen and vitamin D. This is good news for women who want to prevent osteoporosis, arthritis, and other bone-weakening conditions. In one small study published in the *Journal of the Federation of American Societies for Experimental Biology*, 13 postmenopausal women were first fed a diet that provided 0.25 milligrams of boron for 119 days; then they were fed the same diet with a boron supplement of 3 milligrams daily for 48 days. The results revealed that boron supplementation reduced the amount of calcium lost in the urine. This suggests that boron can help prevent osteoporosis, although more research is needed to know for sure.

Next to oxygen, silicon is the most prevalent element on earth. Silicon supports calcium in the maintenance and growth of bones and joints. A UCLA professor, Edith M. Carlisle, Ph.D., found that silicon in the diet of chicks produced denser bone and faster growth compared to chicks deprived of the mineral. Silicon produced a 100 percent increase in the level of collagen, the protein component of bone, which provides the matrix for calcification and imparts flexibility. In rats, it was found that a diet deficient in silicon produced bone deformities and extended the healing time for fractures. The bones of rats given extra silicon were found to contain 20 percent more calcium and 10 percent more phosphorus than those from control rats fed the same diet without the extra silicon.[4] Research will continue on these trace elements to determine their importance for humans.

Estrogen

Estrogen, one of the sex hormones, is integral to the body's efficient use of calcium. Estrogen both increases calcium absorption and decreases its urinary excretion. Any activity or illness that lowers estrogen levels, triggering cessation of menstruation, can bring on significant bone loss, especially from the spine. Very low calorie diets (500 calories), excessive exercise, and anorexia (an eating disorder) are some of these activities. When these activities cause women who are very thin to stop having a menstrual cycle for a year or more, the most bone loss occurs.

The Special Role of Exercise

The bad news is that nearly half of all women 50 and older have low bone mass or osteoporosis—and don't know it. The good news is that regular physical activity maximizes the density of your bones while they are still growing and maturing and then minimizes bone loss later in life. Therefore, the goal for premenopausal women is to build the strongest bone possible during their 20s and early 30s and then maintain this bone from about age 35, when bone building stops, to menopause, when estrogen production declines. Some bone loss is inevitable with age—as early as age 25, women begin losing bone at the rate of 1 percent per year—but it does not have to lead to injury and even death from osteoporosis.

Knowing that calcium won't cure osteoporosis or even prevent bone loss when considered alone, researchers are looking for combinations of factors that can at least slow, if not stop, bone loss. Weight-bearing exercise appears to be one element of the formula.

Bones become stronger with physical stress. If they are not

used, they lose calcium and become porous. In addition, by strengthening the muscles and tendons that protectively surround bone, exercise makes bones less susceptible to injury.

An important study from the Mayo Clinic found that as much as one-half of all spongy bone, like that of the spine, is lost *before* menopause. Weight-bearing exercise such as walking, running, tennis, weight training, and aerobics, is especially effective in stimulating osteoblast growth and building this type of bone in women under age 35.

There's more:

- "Women who exercise twice a week have denser bones than those who exercise once a week, who in turn have denser bones than those who never exercise at all," writes Dr. Whitlock in *The Calcium Plus Workbook*.[5]

- Even sedentary postmenopausal women increased bone mass by 5 percent after nine months of an exercise program and a high-calcium diet.

- Another study found that individuals who walked aerobically retained much more bone mass than those who rode a stationary bicycle or worked out on Nautilus.

Weight-bearing exercises are those that cause your muscles to pull on bones to move some or all of your body or objects you carry through space or against gravity. That means walking, jogging, running, tennis, skiing, hiking, jumping rope, and aerobic dancing. The bone-building effects of lifting weights and trampolining are still being studied. The form of exercise you choose depends on your interests, your physical condition, the cost, and convenience. (It's wise to consult your physician before beginning any exercise program.)

Although research continues to find the optimal exercise

program for bone fitness, Dr. Whitlock makes the following suggestions:

1. Exercise at least three times a week for 20–60 minutes at a low to medium intensity.

2. Activity should be weight-bearing, as described above.

3. Activity should involve pulls on a variety of muscles.

4. Choose activities you enjoy, so you are more likely to continue.

5. Include warm-up and cool-down exercises for about five minutes each—slow stretches and bends that will prepare your muscles for the change of pace.

6. Choose a program that is nontraumatic to your bones and muscles. Consider your physical condition and the shape your bones are in—you don't have to walk four miles the first day.

7. Make sure you have good equipment—well-made walking shoes, for instance. These will help avoid injury and discomfort.

Remember, if you are a premenopausal woman, don't exercise so much that you cause your periods to stop—this causes more harm than good.

THE RISK OF OSTEOPOROSIS

Osteoporosis affects nearly half of women over middle age. The brittle weakening of the bones results, for example, in twice as many women as men suffering hip fractures. The risk factors for developing the disease include:

- **Heredity**—women with female relatives who have osteoporosis are more likely to develop it.

- **Sex**—women's bones are less dense than men's; women tend to take in 50 percent less calcium than men due to food selection and frequent dieting; women live longer than men, so there is more time for the bone loss to take effect (a double-edged sword!).

- **Onset of menopause**—the earlier the onset, the greater the risk of osteoporosis.

- **Ethnic background**—women with ancestors from the British Isles, northern Europe, China, or Japan have the highest risk.

- **Stature and build**—short or medium-height women have a greater risk; slender or excessively thin women have less dense bones than obese women, so feel the bone loss more.

- **Certain diseases**—endocrine disorders, diabetes, and rheumatoid arthritis put women at risk.

- **Cigarette smoking.**

- **Inadequate calcium levels** (as described earlier in this chapter).

- **Inadequate exercise** (see above).

A DIET FOR FIT BONES

The current dietary reference intake (DRI) amounts for women of the several "bone builders" are:

	Calcium (mg)	Phosphorus (mg)	Magnesium (mg)	Boron (mg)*
Over age 25	1,000	1,000	320	1–2
Pregnant	1,200	1,200	320	1–2
Lactating	1,200	1,200	355	1–2

	Vitamin C (mg)	Vitamin D (mcg)	Vitamin K (mcg)
Over age 25	75	5	65
Pregnant	70	10	65
Lactating	95	10	65

Based on data from the Food and Nutrition Board–National Academy of Sciences, 1998.

* Estimates. Values for silicon undetermined.

These nutrients are found in a variety of foods as suggested below.

SOURCES OF BONE-BUILDER NUTRIENTS

CALCIUM

Item	Serving size	Calcium (mg)
Yogurt, plain low-fat	1 cup	415
Sardines, with bones	3 ounces	372
Ricotta, part skim	½ cup	337
Skim milk	1 cup	302
Buttermilk	1 cup	300
Whole sesame seeds	3 tablespoons	300
Whole milk	1 cup	291
Gruyere cheese	1 ounce	287
Swiss cheese	1 ounce	262

Item	Serving size	Calcium (mgs)
Tofu, firm, calcium-fortified	½ cup	258
Turnip greens, cooked	1 cup	250
Bok choy, cooked	1 cup	250
Cheddar cheese	1 ounce	213
Calcium-fortified orange juice	6 ounces	200
Mozzarella cheese, part skim	1 ounce	183
Oysters, raw	¾ cup	170
Salmon, canned with bones	3 ounces	167
Beans, garbanzo, cooked	1 cup	150
Molasses, blackstrap	1 tablespoon	150
Almonds	½ cup	150
Mustard greens, cooked	½ cup	97
Corn muffin	2 medium	90
Cottage cheese, 2 percent fat	½ cup	77
Kale, cooked	½ cup	74
Parmesan cheese, grated	1 tablespoon	69
Broccoli, cooked	½ cup	68
Orange	1 medium	54
Mineral waters (1 liter servings): Contrexeville		451
Mendocino		380
San Pellegrino		200
Perrier		140
Apollinaris		91

Source: Based on data from *Agriculture Handbook* Nos. 8 and 456 (Washington, DC: U.S. Government Printing Office) and other sources.

Phosphorus

Meat, poultry, eggs, fish, dried peas and beans, dairy products, whole grains, carbonated soft drinks

Magnesium
Raw leafy greens, nuts, seeds, whole grains, soybeans

Boron
Fruits and vegetables, especially apples and pears; green leafy vegetables; legumes; nuts

Silicon
Alfalfa, oat bran, wheat bran, soybean meal

Vitamin C
Citrus fruits, melon, strawberries, tomatoes, green peppers, broccoli, Brussels sprouts, potatoes, dark green vegetables

Vitamin D
Fish oils, beef, butter, eggs, fortified nonfat milk, salmon, tuna

Vitamin K
Leafy greens, peas, potatoes, cabbage, liver, cereals

The sample one-week menu plan outlined in Chapter Twelve has been designed to enhance your calcium intake. I've also included a number of hints on ways to increase your dietary calcium effortlessly.

SUPPLEMENTING CALCIUM

Your choices determine how "calcium healthy" you are—you *can* get adequate levels of calcium and its enhancers from your diet by choosing to include some dairy products and a variety of other foods.

However, for postmenopausal women, whose calcium needs some experts believe rise to 1,500 milligrams daily; for pregnant and lactating women; and for any woman who doubts her ability to get a full level of calcium on most days, supplements can be a reassurance.

Supplements should do just that—supplement dietary sources, not replace them. If you have already reviewed your diet (perhaps the food diary described in Chapter Two will help) and estimate that you are getting about 600 milligrams of calcium, then a 200-milligram supplement, not the full 800-milligram daily allowance, will be adequate and safe.

I have described the complex interactions between calcium, its inhibitors, and its enhancers. The bioavailability of the calcium is the key—you are only throwing money away if you take calcium supplements and continue to drink coffee or soft drinks, smoke cigarettes, or avoid exercise. Remove the inhibitors, introduce or increase the enhancers, and then and only then consider your need for supplements (see also Chapter Nine).

Calcium is unstable alone, so supplements must be made with calcium in combination with other minerals. The most common are:

- Calcium carbonate—from oyster shells, with 40 percent calcium

- Calcium citrate—24 percent calcium

- Calcium lactate—from milk sugar (which should be avoided by lactose-intolerant individuals), 13 percent calcium

- Calcium gluconate—9 percent calcium

- Calcium glubionate—6.5 percent calcium

Calcium phosphate contains over 23 percent calcium but is not generally recommended, since our diets tend to have excessive phosphorus. Bone meal (31 percent calcium) and dolomite (22 percent calcium) should also be avoided since they may be contaminated with lead and other toxic minerals.

Studies continue to take place to try to determine which form is most effective. Ralph Shangraw, chairman of the Department of Pharmaceutics at the University of Maryland School of Pharmacy, published the results of his analysis of 80 calcium supplements. He found that almost half of the various brands did not disintegrate and the calcium went unused.[6]

Researchers from the University of Texas Health Sciences Center at Dallas concluded that "calcium citrate provides a more optimum calcium bioavailability than calcium carbonate." Robert Recker, M.D., of Creighton University, Omaha, reported in the *New England Journal of Medicine* that the calcium in citrate form was significantly better absorbed by individuals with low levels of stomach acid (common in women over 40) than was the calcium in the carbonate form.[7]

Use the dietary reference intake chart in the previous section as a guide to your need for supplementation of any or all of the bone builders. Remember, this is not a case for "a little is good, a lot is better." Balance, from varied natural food sources wherever possible, is the key to a lifetime of strong bones.

CHAPTER NINE

Are There "Female" Minerals?

The physician has but a single task: to cure; and if
he succeeds, it matters not a whit by what means he
has succeeded.

—HIPPOCRATES

All of us, men and women alike, are made up of organic
elements—primarily oxygen, carbon, hydrogen, and nitrogen—
and inorganic minerals such as calcium and potassium.
These minerals supply no calories, but they are essential.
Michael Lesser, M.D., in *Nutrition and Vitamin Therapy*, emphasizes, "Humans can tolerate a deficiency of vitamins longer
than a deficiency of minerals. A slight change in the blood's
level of important minerals may rapidly endanger health and
survival."[1]

While it is true, then, that both sexes can feel the effects of
mineral deficiencies, it is also true that women are more likely
to be deficient. The chronic dieter, the nutrition buff, and the
grabber are each in her own way at risk of deficiency.

Richard Kunin, M.D., San Francisco–based author of *Mega-*

Nutrition for Women, writes, "The differences between a man's and a woman's biochemistry are so profound that it is a national scandal that we act as if a woman can be healthy on a male diet.... From month to month, from birth to the giving of life to the change of life, women face a unique challenge to keep their body chemistry in balance."[2]

I believe the answer to the question "Are there 'female' minerals?" has to be yes. They are: calcium, phosphorus, and magnesium, known as bulk or macrominerals because they are present in relatively large quantities in our bodies; and the trace or microminerals (each comprising less than 0.01 percent of our total body weight) iron, zinc, manganese, iodine, and copper. Some of these we have already discussed in detail.

Besides calcium and phosphorus, there is another mineral critical for health. Magnesium is responsible for more biochemical reactions in the body than any other mineral. It tunes up all cells, tissues, and organs—getting the body ready for productive activity and wear and tear. It is the mineral cofactor in DNA cell rebuilding and plays an important role in neuromuscular problems, the cardiac muscle, smooth muscle tissue, nerve impulse transmission, and the metabolism of carbohydrates and amino acids. Magnesium acts as a natural tranquilizer and reduces tremors and cramps. It is a major mineral cofactor in the tranformation of essential fats into prostaglandins, those extraordinarily powerful compounds that control all bodily function on a cellular level.

Magnesium has been found by researchers at the University of California to be low in the blood of many women prior to and during their period. Some women have found it helpful in relieving the symptoms of premenstrual syndrome (see below for more on PMS).

Magnesium appears to be especially important to pregnant women. A classic study published in the British Journal of Obstetrics and Gynecology reports that, compared to a nonsupplemented control group, women given 360 milligrams of supplemental magnesium daily from the third month of pregnancy:[3]

• Were less likely to hemorrhage

• Had fewer cervical problems

• Retained less fluid

• Were more likely to deliver normal-size, responsive babies

Other researchers have found that magnesium levels are low in depressed individuals and rise after recovery. The magnesium in the cells, not in the blood, decreases and may account for the symptoms. Furthermore, low levels of both blood and cellular magnesium have been reported in individuals with high blood pressure.

Women who take the birth control pill should be especially watchful of their magnesium intake, since this medication decreases the mineral in the bloodstream.

Magnesium is the third partner in the bone-building process and is subject to the effects of inhibitors just as calcium and phosphorus are. Preferably, the diet should provide two parts calcium for each part of magnesium. Alcohol; high levels of protein, fat, calcium, phosphorus, or phytic acid; and synthetic vitamin D (as in fortified milk) can negatively affect the mineral's availability within the body.

The DRI for women is:

19 and over	320 milligrams
Pregnant or lactating	300 or 355 milligrams

I personally believe that women need anywhere from 100 milligrams to 1,200 milligrams of magnesium on a daily basis, from supplementation and/or food sources. Food sources include raw leafy greens, sea vegetables, almonds, sunflower seeds, whole grains, blackstrap molasses, and soybeans.

TRACE MINERALS FOR WOMEN

Iron

While our bodies contain only about 4 grams of iron, over half of which is in the red blood cells, it is vital to every tissue in the body. As a component of hemoglobin, it carries oxygen to these tissues. Without it, the oxygen-starved muscles gradually become exhausted and the brain less focused. Symptoms of iron-deficiency anemia include hair loss, pallor, fatigue, forgetfulness, depression, and shortness of breath.

As I detailed in Chapter Four, women are especially prone to iron deficiencies in part because of nature and in part because of the choices we make in diet style. Women lose 2–4 tablespoons of blood each month during menstruation, including 15–30 milligrams of iron. The contraceptive intrauterine device (IUD), by increasing menstrual blood loss, causes even greater iron loss; the birth control pill, by decreasing blood loss, helps retain iron.

Pregnancy further depletes supplies since the mother's blood supplies iron to the fetus. Of course, blood is lost during childbirth, too.

Chronic dieters, who avoid iron-rich meat and eggs out of concern over calories, and nutrition buffs, who avoid them out of concern over cholesterol and saturated fats, are the most likely to be deficient. Since at best only 30 percent of the iron taken in is absorbed, you must eat more than your body needs.

The DRI for women is:

Age 19–50   18 milligrams

Over 50   8 milligrams

Pregnant or lactating   27 or 9 milligrams

Food sources include meat, eggs, leafy greens, beets, kelp, dried beans, enriched cereals and whole grains, pumpkin and sesame seeds, and blackstrap molasses. The herbs yellow dock and dandelion root are additional sources. Cooking in iron pots provides small amounts of this important mineral in your diet as well.

See Chapter Four for more on the virtues of meat and eggs.

Zinc

As a cofactor, zinc is essential for the conversion of the omega-3 and omega-6 oils into prostaglandins. Zinc is essential for body protein synthesis, vitamin metabolism, proper growth, healing of wounds and burns, and development of the sex organs. It promotes the removal of harmful carbon dioxide and is directly involved in the body's metabolism of carbohydrates and energy. It forms part of the insulin component secreted by the pancreas. Zinc helps to enhance digestion, protects the body under stressful conditions, and plays an important role in many major metabolic reactions.

Zinc strengthens hair and nails and helps keep skin unblemished. Deficiencies may cause disruption of menstruation.

The grabber's diet, which emphasizes processed foods, is likely to be zinc deficient since processing removes most zinc found naturally. Nutrition buffs who still follow the high-carbohydrate, low-fat diet popular in the 1990s are also likely to be deficient because the phytic acid in the grains they eat excessively interferes with zinc absorption.

The DRI for women is:

Age 19 and over   15 milligrams

Pregnant   15 milligrams

Lactating   19 milligrams

Food sources include oysters, clams, herring, blackstrap molasses, chicken, beef, sesame and sunflower seeds, liver, bran, whole oatmeal, and wheat germ.

Manganese

Manganese is involved in female sex hormone production; the synthesis of vitamins B, C, and E; and the metabolism of protein, carbohydrates, and fat. Manganese protects bones and ligaments and nourishes the brain and nervous system. The mineral is important in the function of normal reproduction and the mammary glands. Animals that have lost their mothering instinct have been found to be manganese deficient.

Manganese is another mineral that appears to have a role in osteoporosis. Paul Saltman, M.D., at the University of California at San Diego, evaluated blood and bone samples of women with severe osteoporosis and those with no sign of the disease. The osteoporotic women had a manganese level one quarter of the level of the other group. Manganese deficiency is also associated with disk problems and cartilage formation.

The mineral also helps regulate blood sugar levels so that long periods without food will not result in heavy sugar bingeing or a weakening low blood sugar attack. Diabetics, as well as schizophrenics and individuals prone to heart disease and rheumatoid arthritis, are often low in tissue blood levels of manganese.

If either iron or manganese is taken excessively, each may interfere with the other's absorption.

The DRI for women is 2–5 milligrams (more precise levels are not yet known).

Food sources include sea vegetables, buckwheat, whole wheat, barley, brown rice, almonds, beans, peas, and pineapple.

Iodine

Iodine was one of the first minerals recognized as important to human health. Important for healthy breasts, it is also the essential ingredient in the thyroid hormone thyroxine. This hormone controls metabolism, so inadequate supplies can result in fatigue, overweight, and diminished sex drive.

Fifty years ago, people got iodine in their bread—to the tune of 150 micrograms per slice! But, now our breads are made with bromine, a substance that interferes with iodine absorption and can possibly contribute to goiter. So instead of getting a little iodine in your daily bread, you're getting a little bromine, which reduces your iodine levels further.

Low levels of iodine can disrupt the breakdown of estrogen, resulting in excess estrogen and the problems it can cause. Deficiencies may also cause dry hair and skin.

Conversely, iodine has been shown helpful in fibrocystic breast disease and as an expectorant. In the levels found in cough syrups, however, it worsens acne.

The DRI for women is:

Age 19 and over   150 micrograms

Pregnant   175 micrograms

Lactating   200 micrograms

Food sources include sea vegetables, kelp, sea salt, herring, seafood, cod liver oil, and vegetables grown in iodine-rich soil.

Copper

When everything is in balance, we have just a pinch of copper in our bodies. Yet it is essential for incorporating iron into hemoglobin; forming melanin for skin color and collagen for strong bones, joints, and connective tissue; and synthesizing neurotransmitters to carry impulses throughout the nervous system. Several enzymes need copper to build body tissue, and it contributes to fertility and completion of pregnancy. Copper aids in resistance to infection and retention of calcium in bones.

Copper is abundant in today's environment, so few women are technically deficient. More commonly, problems arise with imbalances in the delicate system of copper synthesis, resulting in biounavailable, unbound, and ultimately toxic copper.

Copper plumbing and cookware contribute to our copper load, as does the drinking water in some areas. The birth control pill tends to raise blood copper levels, and some experts believe copper may be absorbed from copper IUDs.

Our diet may contribute as well. Copper is an effective fungicide, so copper sulfate may be sprayed on fruits and vegetables. Soybeans and tofu, staples in the vegetarian diet, are naturally high in copper, as are oysters, calf and lamb liver, and regular tea.

Several physiological conditions affect copper usage and accumulation, the most important being the activity of the adrenal gland. When the adrenal gland malfunctions from stress—too much sugar or caffeine, alcohol, or tobacco—it causes ceruloplasmin production to slow down in the liver. Since about 95 percent of the copper in our blood is bound to ceruloplasmin, a prerequisite to copper use, without it unbound copper accumulates in the brain, liver, and other organs.

Zinc, which ideally should be present in a ratio of 8:1 with copper, helps prevent copper accumulation. However, with decreased consumption of zinc-rich meat and eggs and increased consumption of zinc-inhibiting sugars and grains, zinc deficiencies are common. In addition, sudden stress simultaneously raises blood copper levels and lowers blood zinc.

When copper is stored and not used, problems arise. High blood or tissue copper levels have been associated with:

- Acne
- Hair loss
- Anemia
- Rheumatoid arthritis
- Premenstrual syndrome (PMS)
- Osteoporosis
- Candidiasis (yeast infections)
- Elevated estrogen levels
- Decreased sexual function
- Various nervous disorders, including depression, phobias, and schizophrenia

Blood tests can determine copper levels. Tissue mineral analysis (hair analysis) is another effective way to measure copper levels as well as a variety of heavy metals. (Visit www. unikeyhealth.com.)

Several vitamins and minerals are known to lower copper levels by binding with it to pull it out of storage or to carry it out of the body. These include the vitamins B_6, C, folic acid, and niacin (B_3) and the minerals sulfur, molybdenum, iron, manganese, and zinc.

My diet plan outlined in the remaining chapters can help maintain the effective copper balance: it retains zinc-rich meat and eggs, monitors the copper-rich grains, and avoids the stressors sugars and caffeine.

The DRI for women is 2 milligrams.

Food sources include liver, kidneys, oysters, wheat germ, soybeans, mushrooms, blackstrap molasses, dried beans, and nuts.

PMS: A DEFICIENCY DISORDER?

There is a condition from which 70–90 percent of American women of childbearing age suffer ... a condition that disrupts lives, causes recurring pain and suffering, and may even bring on violence and death ... a condition that may have afflicted Queen Victoria and Mary Todd Lincoln ... a condition for which there are no diagnostic tests, no clearly defined cause, no definitive cure ... a condition called premenstrual syndrome, or just PMS.

What does PMS have to do with "female" minerals? Almost all of the minerals I have discussed (and a few others) have a role in various symptoms of PMS and, therefore, in therapy (see chart). In fact, nutritional imbalance and its integral role with hormonal imbalance may one day prove to be a key to unlocking this Pandora's box.

NUTRIENT DEFICIENCIES AND PMS

Nutrient	Status at Menstruation	Effects
B$_6$ (pyridoxine)	Deficient prior to	Mood swings
Calcium	Lower prior to	Muscle cramps, pelvic pain, bloating, nervousness
Magnesium	May be lower prior to	Cravings, mood swings, bloating, breast tenderness
Zinc	May be deficient	Headaches, irritability, depression or nervousness, cramps
Iron	May be deficient	Anemia, fatigue, weakness
Potassium	May be deficient	Fluid retention, headaches, tiredness
Sodium	Elevated	Weight gain, bloating
Copper	Elevated	Reduced adrenal activity, deficiencies in other minerals, depression
Vitamin E	May be deficient	Fluid retention, cramps, breast tenderness

While many women experience menstrual cramping, headaches, or low back pain during their period, PMS generally refers to the symptoms that occur 1–10 days prior to menstruation. These symptoms usually improve once menstruation begins. Most women have more than one symptom, but they usually experience the same cluster month after month.

Researcher Guy Abraham, M.D., has divided the symptoms into four subclasses, based on their most common groupings among women:[4]

PMS A (Anxiety): 65–75 percent of sufferers

- Nervous tension
- Mood swings
- Irritability
- Anxiety

Vitamin B_6 and magnesium are particularly helpful.

PMS H (Heavy): 50–65 percent of sufferers

- Weight gain
- Swelling of hands and feet
- Abdominal bloating
- Breast tenderness

Magnesium, vitamin B_6, and vitamin E may help relieve symptoms.

PMS C (Craving): 25–35 percent of sufferers

- Headache
- Craving for sweets or salty foods
- Increased appetite
- Dizziness or fainting spells
- Fatigue

Vitamins B_6 and C, zinc, and GLA can help.

PMS D (Depression): 25–35 percent of sufferers

- Depression
- Forgetfulness
- Crying
- Confusion
- Insomnia

Magnesium and essential fatty acids (EFAs) help some women.

The underlying cause or causes of PMS are not yet known. Several researchers, including Katharina Dalton of England, suspect an imbalance in the estrogen-progesterone ratio with excessive levels of estrogen, a condition known as estrogen dominance. Furthermore, citing an apparent deficiency in EFAs among premenstrual women, some experts postulate that without adequate EFAs, the body will not produce enough prostaglandin E1. This substance in turn has a controlling effect on the female hormone prolactin and complex interactions with steroids. Further supporting this theory is the known role that magnesium, zinc, and vitamins B_3, B_6, and C have in the conversion of EFAs to PGE1 (see Chapter Three).

Optimizing production of the prostaglandins from EFAs is central to the plan I recommend to my clients and describe in this book. In addition, the plan's emphasis on avoiding caffeine, sugar, and excess sodium is a built-in prescription for relief from PMS. Only when we choose health, when we take back control of our diets, will we control our hormones, not the other way around.

SUPER FEMALE FOODS

In Chapter Ten, I give a staples shopping list for foods that will help ensure long-term health and fitness. However, because of their abundance of "female" minerals and other vitamins and minerals essential to every woman's good looks and health, I have designated some foods as Super Female Foods. Here's my list, along with the significant nutrients they contain:

- **Blackstrap molasses** (residue from sugar refining)—vitamins B_1, B_2, inositol, PABA; iron, calcium, magnesium, potassium, copper, chromium, molybdenum

- **Brewer's yeast** (dried yeast derived from brewing beer and ale)—vitamins B_1, B_2, B_3, B_6, B_{15}, folic acid, biotin, choline, PABA; iron, calcium, phosphorus, potassium, zinc, selenium, chromium (Note: Moderation is essential with this one, since too much may encourage candida overgrowth.)

- **Broccoli**—vitamins A (beta-carotene), C, folic acid; iron, calcium, selenium

- **Brown rice**—vitamins B_3, B_6, B_{15}, pantothenic acid, folic acid, biotin, choline; magnesium, manganese, selenium

- **Grass-fed red meat**—protein, minerals, vitamin B_{12}, vitamin A, vitamin D, omega-3 fats, and CLA

- **Ground or milled flaxseeds and flaxseed oil**—omega-3 fatty acids galore. The seeds contain high amounts of soluble and insoluble fiber; they are the richest source of lignans—plant-based estrogen modulators—and they also contain protein, vitamins, and minerals

- **Lentils**—vitamins B_1, B_6, pantothenic acid, folic acid, biotin, choline, inositol; iron, calcium, potassium

- **Fatty fish**—protein, omega-3 fatty acids (especially EPA and DHA)

- **Omega-3 eggs**—essential fatty acids (especially DHA), vitamin E, vitamin B_{12}, antioxidants including lutein

- **Pure unsweetened cranberry juice**—flavonoids, enzymes, and organic acids such as malic acid, citric acid, and quinic acid

- **Sea vegetables**—vitamins A, B_1, B_2, B_3, B_{12}; calcium, magnesium, potassium, iodine, selenium, chromium, molybdenum, vanadium, lithium, silicon

- **Sesame seeds**—vitamins B_1, B_3, B_{15}, B_{17}; zinc, potassium, phosphorus, calcium, iron; EFAs

- **Sunflower seeds**—vitamins B_1, B_3, pantothenic acid, PABA; magnesium, potassium, zinc; EFAs

Nutritional Treasures from the Sea

One item on the list of Super Female Foods is not yet familiar to many Americans: sea vegetables. Although they have an ancient past, sea vegetables are of particular interest today to women who want to ensure good health.

Sea vegetables have absorbed nutrients from the sea via not just their roots but also their leaves and stems. As the list above indicates, they are chock full of hard-to-find trace minerals, as well as the more common calcium and iron (10 times more than spinach). Here is a brief rundown on the more commonly available types, with suggestions for preparation:

- **Hijiki**—tastes a bit like licorice and looks like tangled black strings; contains 14 times the calcium in a glass of cow's milk. Rinse in cold water, then soak for 20 minutes. Hijiki can be added to soups or salads; it is delicious sautéed with carrots and fresh ginger.

- **Wakame**—a delicately flavored dark green leaf. Rinse in cold water, soak for 15 minutes. Add to soups, on top of fish, or in dressings.

- **Kombu**—a kelp with a sweet/salty flavor. It can be toasted in the oven for snacks, added to beans (aids digestion), or crumbled and sprinkled over fish, chicken, or rice dishes. Cut into strips, it can be added to soups.

- **Nori** (green laver or sea lettuce)—a nutty-tasting seaweed, high in B_{12} and A, that comes in sheets. It can be toasted and crumbled over vegetables, pasta, or fish. Or use it untoasted to wrap other foods.

- **Arame**—a taste and appearance similar to hijiki. Rinse in cool water, then soak for 10–15 minutes; it more than doubles in size. Add to salads, soups, brown rice, and vegetables. Both hijiki and arame can also be sautéed for 2–3 minutes in oil.

- **Agar agar**—a seaweed that is sold in flake form to be used in place of gelatin for thickening puddings, molds, and mousses.

A WORD ABOUT SUPPLEMENTS

Americans currently spend over $3 billion annually on vitamin and mineral supplements. Clearly, millions of men and women think they are getting some value; however, the experts don't always agree among themselves whether or not this is true.

Over twenty years ago, when the American Medical Association (AMA) reviewed the issue of vitamin supplements, it concluded that normal, healthy people receive adequate nutrition from their diet and do not need to take vitamins. Even though there was a great deal of evidence in favor of vitamin supplements, long-term double-blind nutrition studies were just beginning.

In the past five years, the results of those long-term studies have shown the health benefits of vitamins. The medical journals have published reports that helped establish minimum daily requirements and provided proof that vitamins can actually reduce the incidence of certain chronic diseases.

In 2002, the AMA announced that, based on the results of these long-term clinical studies, it has *reversed* its previous position regarding supplementation. Now the AMA recommends that everyone take a multivitamin supplement every day.

Supplements cannot and should not replace food. The delicate mineral balance needed for effective calcium utilization highlights the kind of chemistry nature provides—broccoli is a source not just of calcium, but also of beta-carotene, vitamin C, iron, folic acid, and fiber. Imbalances can quickly arise if a single mineral is emphasized in supplements.

Nevertheless, most women will benefit from some supplementation. Environmental pollutants deplete nutrients from our bodies through the process of detoxification and elimination. Medications such as aspirin cancel out nutrients; birth control pills cause deficiencies of folic acid and vitamins B_6 and B_{12}. Topsoil depletion, food processing, and storage time decrease the levels of nutrients contained in foods.

Certain events in women's lives, such as pregnancy, lactation, and menopause, put such demands on our bodies that even the 3 percent of us who eat appropriate amounts from all the food groups are unlikely to meet our bodies' needs.

I would suggest that, given widespread deficiencies of zinc and magnesium and the need for these and other nutrients in the conversion of EFAs to the protective prostaglandins, women should take a multivitamin and mineral supplement containing the vitamins niacin (B_3), B_6, C, and E; the antioxidant beta-carotene; and the minerals zinc, magnesium, and selenium.

Choosing especially nutrient-rich foods and supplementing key nutrients can help you feel and look better. If modern science can allow many of us to live longer than was thought possible just 50 or 100 years ago, then our responsibility to ourselves to make our later years healthy years is a great one. The following chapters outline my plan for us to take control of our health destiny.

CHAPTER TEN

What to Eat, How to Heat

Eat . . . and be healthy.
—MY GRANDMOTHER CLARA

LABEL READING: WORTH THE EFFORT

Since the average supermarket may contain over 30,000 items (with nearly 8,000 new food products entering the marketplace each year), label reading is a necessity. It is a fairly simple task to decode any food label once you understand the rules of the game.

The basic rule is that the Food and Drug Administration requires food manufacturers to list ingredients of greatest amount by descending order of weight. This means that if a "natural" or "lite" oatmeal cookie, for example, lists apple juice concentrate (which contains fructose, a fruit sugar) as the first ingredient, then the cookie contains more concentrate than any other ingredient, including oats.

If a product carries a health claim, then additional information is also provided, such as calories; grams of protein, fat, and sodium; and vitamin and mineral content per serving. Manufacturers must now list dietary fiber and cholesterol grams for concerned consumers.

Fat Finding

When it comes to identifying fat, the FDA-required food labels have come a long way. Ten years ago, a food label was only required to list the amount of fat by weight. So, for example, we learned that 2 percent milk contained 2 percent of fat by weight. Now, we can easily spot the amount of fat by calories and we have learned that that same milk is actually 36 percent fat by calories.

In addition, for every food, the FDA requires a listing of the calories from saturated fat and the amount of cholesterol. It has also defined certain fat-related terms to help us know what we are buying:

- **Fat-free** products contain "trivial" amounts of fat, less than 0.5 mg per serving.

- **Low-fat** products contain 3 grams of fat or less per serving.

- **Low-saturated fat** foods provide no more than 1 gram of saturated fat per serving.

- **Reduced-fat** products must contain at least 25 percent less fat than the regular version of the same food.

- **"Light"** foods must contain one-third fewer calories and/ or one-half the fat of the original version.

- **"Healthy"** foods must meet the qualifications for low-fat and low-saturated fat. They must also contain only limited amounts of cholesterol and sodium.

All this attention to the amount of fat in foods may seem comforting to many consumers. And it's true that knowledge is power when it comes to making wise purchases at the grocery store. Unfortunately, when it comes to fat, food labels remain focused on the wrong issue.

I have always maintained that the amount of fat we consume is less important than the type of fat in our foods. Food labels are required only to list the total fat and the amount of saturated fat. This vilifies saturated fat, leading consumers to believe that it is inherently harmful. While some manufacturers voluntarily list the amount of monounsaturated and polyunsaturated fat, a key piece of information—the amount of trans fat—is missing!

As of January 1, 2006, labels will have to list the trans fat content. For foods that contain trans fat, an asterisk at the end of "saturated fat" will direct consumers to a footnote indicating how much of this amount is trans fat. Foods without trans fat may make the nutritional claim, "Trans Fat Free." Implementation of this new ruling may take some time as food manufacturers transition to the new label requirements, but many are removing trans fats from their foods already and even restaurants are getting in on the act.

In the meantime, how can you tell if a product contains trans fat? One clue is to look for the words "hydrogenated" or "partially hydrogenated" in the list of ingredients. While this won't tell you how much trans fat is in the food, you can take an educated guess. Remember that the list of ingredients on labels is in order from most prevalent by weight to least prevalent. So, the higher hydrogenated fat is on the list, the more trans fat in the product.

Another method, while not foolproof, is to add up the numbers for the types of fat listed on the label. If they do not equal the amount of total fat, the "missing link" may well be trans fat. This only works if a label lists all three fats—saturated, monounsaturated, and polyunsaturated. Look at the total fat grams and subtract all the listed fats. The difference is trans fat grams. For example, if a food label lists 10 grams of total fat per serving, with 2 grams saturated fat, 5 grams polyunsaturated fat, and 2 grams monounsaturated fat, the three fats total 9 grams (2 + 5 + 2 = 9). Take the 10 grams of total fat and subtract the 9 grams listed and the difference is 1 gram. Now you know that this food has 1 gram of trans fat per serving.

Trans fat is found in foods containing shortening, including pastries and fried foods, but also turns up in places you might not expect, such as cereals and waffles. So, as you shop, be mindful of the type of fat in each food you buy. Aim for a large "dose" of the healthy essential fats and avoid those poisonous trans fats.

For more information on FDA guidelines, visit www.fda.gov.

Searching for Salt

It is unfortunate that all salt has gotten a bad reputation because of the detrimental effects of refined table salt. Table salt is an unbalanced salt excessively high in sodium chloride and stripped of its other essential trace minerals like magnesium, bromine, and sulfur. In proper mineral balance, natural salt is used by the body to cleanse mucous membranes, regulate body fluids, and normalize blood pressure. Not only is commercial table salt minerally unbalanced, it also contains a number of chemical additives, such as bleaches, conditioners, and anticaking agents, which are toxic to our systems. In fact, sodium chloride in an unadulterated, pure form may very well be the most vital element contained in blood plasma.

When salt is refined and combined with other chemical additives, its metabolic functions are changed. Refined salt does not dissolve in the body; it hardens, leaving deposits in organs and tissue that can result in arterial plaque buildup. Any salt can be tested for its metabolic acceptability by adding 2 tablespoonfuls to a glass of plain water and letting it stand for a couple of hours. If no residue remains on the bottom of the glass, then the salt will dissolve in the fluids of the body as well. If residue remains, this signals unbalanced processed substances unfit for human consumption.

Sea salts are commercially available. Yet these salts can also be refined and may contain chemical pollutants from waste materials in our oceans.

Proper salt intake is essential, especially in summer and for athletes, because so much of the mineral leaves the body fluids via perspiration, tears, and urine.

The USDA Food Guidelines suggest that 1,100–2,400 milligrams per day is a safe sodium intake for most adults. Many women, particularly those with high blood pressure or who retain fluid and bloat easily, need to watch salt intake more carefully. If you are one of these women, consider reducing your total sodium intake to about 1,500 milligrams (¾ teaspoon).

Since most of the salt in our diets comes from canned, bottled, frozen, and processed or fast foods, you will have to learn to decipher the various disguises of salt listed on food labels. When eating in fast-food restaurants, be aware that one chicken breast from Kentucky Fried Chicken contains 1,116 milligrams of sodium, McDonald's Big Mac delivers 1,070 milligrams, and its Egg McMuffin can add 710 milligrams to your diet. A Taco Bell taco is one of your best bets at 280 milligrams. (Note that as in all fast foods, no matter what the sodium level, you still may be getting too much of the wrong kinds of fats.)

To reduce sodium in your diet, try to avoid or cut down on the following:

- Snacks: chips, pretzels, crackers, dips

- Condiments: soy sauce, tamari, mustard, catsup, miso, ca-
pers, barbecue sauce, chili sauce, salad dressings, Worcestershire sauce, meat tenderizers, bouillon cubes, pickles,
monosodium glutamate (MSG); onion, celery, or garlic
salts (powders are all right)

- Cured meats: hot dogs, luncheon meats, sausages, bacon

- Sauerkraut

- Cheese

- Canned fish and vegetables

- Self-rising white flour

Fortunately, many food items are now available in either
"salt-free" or "sodium-restricted" forms. Later in this chapter
I provide a listing of healthy foods in convenient packages.

Label ingredient listings that include baking powder, baking soda, sodium propionate (a mold inhibitor), sodium ben-
zoate (a preservative), or other sodium derivatives (look for
the -ate ending), no matter what their purpose, indicate high
levels of sodium and are a warning signal. You can further cut
down by choosing foods that are naturally low in sodium, including most fruits and vegetables, or that are labeled "very low
sodium," which by law means a sodium content of 35 milligrams or less per serving.

There are several ways to add flavor without salt, some of
which are given later in this chapter. I give additional tips in
Chapter Twelve about using herbs, spices, flavor extracts, and
alcohol in cooking to create taste without added salt.

Another way to control sodium at the table is by seasoning
after cooking. Research has shown that salt added after cooking

tastes stronger than when added before or during cooking. Remember, however, when you add salt that:

¼ teaspoon = 500 milligrams sodium
½ teaspoon = 1,000 milligrams
¾ teaspoon = 1,500 milligrams
1 teaspoon = 2,000 milligrams

Kelp powder, a seaweed powder, can be used in place of salt. Used in one-half the quantities of regular salt, kelp contains a potassium-sodium ratio of 3:1, which more resembles that contained in body fluids (5:1) than does salt (1:10,000).

Stalking Sugar

Most of our dietary intake of sugar (about 156 pounds per person per year) is hidden in packaged foods. Watch out for all sugar sources, and keep in mind that up to five different kinds of sugar can be listed for one product. It all adds up. The following names mean sugar to your body, no matter how you spell them:

• Juice concentrate: apple, pear, peach, pineapple

• Sucrose, dextrose, lactose, maltose, fructose

• Corn sweetener

• Barley or corn malt

• Syrup: corn, rice, maple, malt

• Sugar: invert, brown, raw

• Honey

Mannitol, sorbitol, and xylitol are considered sugar substitutes. They are actually sugar-based alcohols. Found mainly in sugar-free gums, candies, and baked goods for diabetics, they all contain both calories and carbohydrates and have been known to cause diarrhea in sensitive individuals.

Abandoning Aluminum

Label reading is also a way to prevent aluminum from entering your diet; your ultimate goal is to eliminate aluminum entirely from your food. Check ingredient listings for aluminum frequently used in salt, baking powder (unless label specifies nonaluminum baking powder), cake mixes, self-rising flour, processed American cheese, nondairy creamers, and pickled fruits and vegetables. Soft drinks (which are not recommended because of their bone-robbing phosphoric acid content) will add unwanted aluminum to your diet if they are packaged in aluminum cans. The same goes for many types of beer and mineral water.

Many waxed cardboard beverage containers, especially for juices, are lined with aluminum. The acidic fruits and vegetables leach the metal into the food.

Nonfood items, such as antacids, vaginal douches, and antidiarrhetics, can also contain this heavy metal. Substitute products without aluminum.

CONFESSIONS OF A FAST-FOOD NUTRITIONIST

Fast-food nutrition is no longer a contradiction in terms. Over the years I have discovered many shortcuts to wholesome foods without shortchanging nutrition. Like so many women, I am constantly on the go and have had to translate the concerns of the chronic dieter, nutrition buff, and grabber into fit but fast foods.

It is also true that, by nature, I really don't like to cook ... but I do love to eat, so healthy convenience foods are doubly important to me. I also favor eating organically grown produce and meats and poultry raised without artificial hormones or antibiotics. Based on our hectic lifestyles and desire to eat "safe" foods, I have developed a list of food staples that you may find helpful whether at home or on the road.

I am providing this list with brand names for easier shopping. Many of these foods can currently be found in the health food section of a well-stocked supermarket or at your natural food store or food cooperative. Since increasing numbers of food retailers are concerned about the consumer's rising interest in pesticide- and preservative-free food, you may find your local store manager receptive to your suggestions of products to stock.

This list features packaged, jarred, or canned foods. A complete shopping list for total nutrition appears later in this chapter.

Healthy Foods in Convenient Packages

DAIRY PRODUCTS
Continental, Colombo, and Dannon yogurts
Altadena, Friendship or Old Home 2% cottage cheese
Calabro ricotta cheese
Horizon or Nancy's Swiss, Gruyere, mozzarella, mild cheddar, and Monterey Jack. (One ounce of these cheeses provides from 180 to 280 milligrams of calcium. Even 1 tablespoon of Parmesan cheese offers 69 milligrams of calcium.)
Unikey Fat Flush Whey

FAST FIXES (SIDE DISHES, APPETIZERS, SNACKS)
Arrowhead Mills Quick Brown Rice
Barbara's Instant Mashed Potatoes
Ancient Harvest Quinoa Elbow Pasta
Lotus Foods Forbidden Rice and Bhutanese Red Rice
Fantastic Foods Fantastic Falafel or Tabouli
Lundberg RizCous (like couscous, only rice), Cajun or French
    Country Herb Style
Nile Spice Couscous Salad Mix, Basmati Rice, and Red Lentils
Carmel Kosher Potato Pancake or Kugel Mixes
Health Valley Lentil Pilaf, Amaranth Pilaf, Jalapeño Bean Dip,
    Onion Bean Dip, Taco Dip, Taco Sauce
Rice Tech Pastariso Pastas (100% rice)
Vita-spelt Whole Spelt Pasta

CANNED FOODS
Water-packed tuna, salmon, and sardines
Water chestnuts
Chun King Chinese Vegetables
Ortega Chilies
Black pitted olives (rinse under running water)
Muir Glen Tomato Puree, Sauce, Paste, and Whole Peeled
    Tomatoes

SOUPS
Hain Turkey Rice, Minestrone, Vegetable Chicken, Italian Vege-
    table, Italian Vege-pasta
Health Valley Split Pea, Chicken Broth, Beef Broth
Shelton's Chicken Broth

FROZEN FOODS
Northwest Natural Salmon Medallions
Health Valley Turkey or Chicken Wieners (nitrate free)

Shelton's Turkey Breakfast Sausage (nitrate free)
Bounty of the Sea Tuna Franks
Cascadian Farms strawberries or raspberries, green beans, or
    cauliflower (organic)
Nature's Hilights Organic Brown Rice Pizza Crust

CEREALS
American Prairie hot and cold cereals (organic)
Kolln Oat Bran Crunch
Kashi 5 Bran Instant Cereal
Lundberg Creamy Rice (organic)
Pocono Cream of Buckwheat

BREADS, CRACKERS, TORTILLAS, AND TACO SHELLS
French Meadows Woman's Bread
French Meadows Men's Bread
French Meadow Healthseed Spelt Bread
Rainier's Sprouted 16 Grain and Seed Bread
Rainier's Ezekiel 4:9 Bread
Bran A Crisp
Fiber Rich Bran Crackers
Garden of Eatin blue corn tortillas and corn tortillas (organic)
Fiber Crisp rye crackers
Ry Vita
Lifestream Wheat and Rye Krispbread (organic)
Wasa Crispbread hearty and golden rye
Finn crisp rye
Kavli rye
Nejaimes Lavasch (Armenian crackerbread)
Little Bear blue corn and corn taco shells (organic)

SNACKS

Nuts, unshelled: almonds, walnuts, filberts, and peanuts
Good Health Natural Foods Olive Oil Potato Chips
Seeds: sunflower, sesame, and pumpkin
Ralph's Low-Salt Bavarian Pretzels
Popcorn (air-popped)
Terra Sweet Potato Chips
Arrowhead Mills Deaf Smith Peanut Butter (organic)
The Bean Chip (salted or unsalted)
Westbrae Almond Butter
Arrowhead Mills Sesame Tahini (organic)
Shelton's Beef and Turkey Jerky

CONDIMENTS

Spectrum Natural Organic Mayonnaise
Dijon salt-free mustard
Westbrae Sugar-free Unketchup
Enrico's Spaghetti Sauce with Mushrooms
Tree of Life No-Salt-Added Pasta Sauce or Salsa (organic)
New England Organic Dill Pickles (no salt)
Rosarita Enchilada Sauce
Balsamic or raspberry vinegar
Vanilla extract
Variety of dried herbs and nonirradiated spices: garlic powder,
    onion powder, dill, cumin, parsley, dried mustard, basil,
    cinnamon, oregano, rosemary, ginger, tumeric, cloves
Real Salt

BEVERAGES

Sparkling mineral waters
Penta water
Filtered water

Water with lemon or lime
Frey wines (organic)
Domaine de la Busque wines (organic)
Dandelion root tea
Assorted herbal teas
Pau d'arco or taheebo herb tea (thought by some to be bene-
    ficial to candida sufferers)
Teeccino herbal coffee (I keep this on hand for guests, since I
    don't drink coffee)
Mountain Sun or Knudsen's Pure Unsweetened Cranberry
    Juice
V-8 Juice
Muir Glen 100% Vegetable Juice

SWEET TREATS
Pamela's Products gourmet wheat-free and gluten-free cook-
    ies and biscotti
Lifestream Essene fruit cake, raisin, pumpernickel-rye, seed,
    multigrain, cinnamon-date, rye seed, and muffins (great
    toasted plain)

A NOTE ABOUT PESTICIDES
AND FOOD IRRADIATION

While taste, convenience, and nutrition are important factors
in selecting foods, women are also concerned about the overuse
of pesticides in America's food supply.

I urge you to protect yourself and your family by looking
for organic produce (check your local health food store or
food cooperative, as well as increasing numbers of super-

markets), buying domestically grown fruits and vegetables in season (imported produce can contain pesticides banned in the United States), and growing your own foods in gardens or planter boxes.

Exposing foods to radiation leaves very dangerous residues. The group Food and Water can provide you with information on what you can do to stop radiation-exposed food. Call 1-800-EAT-SAFE.

I have also been concerned about the growing number of both chemicals and parasites in America's food supply for many years. The use of insecticides, fungicides, and weed killers is over double that of 30 years ago—over 1 billion pounds of these chemicals per year.

Below is the detoxifying cleansing bath that I use for all kinds of foods: fruits, vegetables, beef, poultry, eggs, fish, and shellfish. It has been used successfully by my patients for over 20 years.

1. Use ½ teaspoon Clorox bleach to 1 gallon of water, obtained from your usual source. Only the Clorox brand will work, so do not substitute any other product.

2. Place the foods to be treated into the bath according to the chart below. Make a separate bath for each group.

3. Remove foods from the Clorox bath and place in clear water for 10 minutes. Dry all foods thoroughly and store.

FOOD CLEANSING SCHEDULE

Food group	Treatment time
Vegetables, leafy	15 minutes
Vegetables, root, thick-skinned, or fibrous	30 minutes
Fruits, thin-skinned berries, peaches, apricots, plums	15 minutes
Fruits, thick-skinned such as apples, citrus, and bananas	30 minutes
Chicken, fish, meats, eggs	20 minutes

Note: Meats can be thawed in a Clorox bath. The timing is about 20 minutes for a weight of 2 to 5 pounds. Frozen turkey or chicken should remain in the Clorox bath until thawed. Ground meats, of course, cannot undergo this process.

ALERT: If you suspect your food has been irradiated, first clean food with a solution of 2 tablespoons of baking soda to 1 gallon of water and leave for 20 minutes. Then place in clear water for 10 minutes. Continue with Clorox bath program as outlined. Most chicken and potatoes are now irradiated.

THE COMPLETE KITCHEN OF THE 21ST CENTURY: A GUIDE TO STOCKING AND SERVING PORTIONS

Throughout this book, I have made suggestions for foods to eat or to avoid. Here it is, all put together to give you a guide to selecting foods that will help you avoid deficiencies, especially zinc, calcium, magnesium, iron, phosphorus, potassium, and the B vitamins.

Essential and Healthy Fats

Choose from a variety of healthy and essential fat sources. Look for the words "organic" and "100 percent expeller-pressed" on the label. Health From The Sun makes a wide variety of healthful oils and is a strong advocate of educating the consumer on the importance of oils in the diet. One to 2 tablespoons of oil a day, either as pure oil or from any of the food sources listed below, is all it takes for healthy skin, hair, and nails, and good reproductive health. Even cholesterol management is enhanced by using the right oils.

Oils to choose from include flaxseed, macadamia, sesame, pumpkin seed, peanut, avocado, olive, hazelnut, walnut, rice bran, almond, high-oleic safflower, and high-oleic sunflower. Mayonnaise, made from expeller-pressed oil, is also a good source.

Each food source listed below is broken down to equal the equivalent of 1 teaspoon of oil (e.g. 1 tablespoon of pumpkin seeds or of mayonnaise equals 1 teaspoon of pure oil).

NUTS (ALL RAW OR HOME-TOASTED IN OVEN)

Nut	Amount
Almonds	7
Brazil nuts	2 medium
Cashews	4–5
Hazelnuts (filberts)	5
Macadamia nuts	3
Pecans	5 halves
Pine nuts (pignoli)	1 tablespoon
Pistachios	15
Walnuts	4 halves

Seeds (raw or home-toasted, 1 tablespoon): flax, pumpkin, sunflower, squash, and sesame, among others

Many of the natural oils have a distinct flavor, making some better for salads, others for sautéeing. This chart will help you select the best oil for each method.

OIL SELECTION BY COOKING METHOD

Oil	Cooking	Baking	Frying	Sautéeing	Sauces	Salads
Flaxseed					X	X
Macadamia	X	X	X	X	X	X
Olive, pure	X			X	X	X
Olive, extra-virgin	X			X	X	X
Peanut	X			X	X	
High-oleic safflower	X	X	X			X
Sesame	X	X		X	X	X
High-oleic sunflower	X	X	X			

Vegetables

A portion equals ½ cup cooked or 1 cup raw, unless otherwise indicated. Of special interest to women are calcium-rich vegetables like bok choy, broccoli, kale, and sea vegetables. Try to eat colorfully for all-around nutrition: orange and yellow foods feature vitamins A and C, red and blue foods (like beets and seaweeds) give us iron, and green foods highlight magnesium and vitamin A. They are all valuable sources of dietary fiber; each serving contains between 2 and 3 grams of fiber. At least four colorful servings of vegetables and fruits are suggested daily. Note: Frequent intake of greens from beets, dandelion, mustard, turnips, as well as spinach and sorrel, should be limited because of the calcium-inhibiting effects of oxalic acid.

Artichoke (½ large, cooked)
Asparagus
Beans (both green and yellow)
Beets
Bok choy (Chinese chard or
    white mustard cabbage)
Broccoli
Brussels sprouts
Cabbage
Carrots
Carrot juice (¼ cup or 2 fluid
    ounces)
Cauliflower
Celery
Cilantro (coriander or Chinese
    parsley)
Chicory
Chilies
Chinese cabbage (napa)
Cucumber
Daikon (long white radish)
Eggplant
Endive
Escarole
Garlic

Greens (collard, radicchio,
    arugula, mache)
Jerusalem artichoke
    (sunchoke)
Jicama
Kale
Lettuce (romaine, bibb,
    Boston)
Mushrooms
Okra
Onions
Parsley
Peppers (all colors)
Radishes
Rutabaga
Snow peas (Chinese pea pods)
Spinach
Sprouts (alfalfa, radish, mung
    bean, clover, adzuki)
Squash (yellow or crookneck,
    Italian or zucchini,
    spaghetti, chayote)
Tomatoes
Vegetable juice (½ cup)
Watercress
Water chestnuts (6 whole)

Sea vegetables: Eden has the widest variety of packaged sea vegetables available, including nori, hijiki, kombu, and arame. Particularly rich in calcium and iron, they can be used in soups, as edible garnishes, or as side dishes. Nutrient information and some suggested cooking tips are included in Chapter Nine.

Fruits

Since many women overdo fruits in the mistaken belief that because they are natural they can be eaten without limits, suggested portions are indicated to help you monitor your intake. Each portion contains about 2 grams of fiber. Remember at least five servings of fruits and vegetables are recommended daily. If candida is out of control, the sugar from fruits should be substantially reduced (just one fruit a day) or even temporarily avoided. Keep in mind that eating the fresh fruit itself, rather than in juice form, provides dietary fiber and is more filling. The fruits listed here are all fresh, sun-dried, or packed without sugar or syrup.

Fruit	Serving portion
Apple	1 small (2-inch diameter)
Apple butter (sugar free)	2 tablespoons
Apple juice or cider	1/3 cup
Applesauce (unsweetened)	1/2 cup
Apricots (fresh)	2 medium
Apricots (dried)	4 halves
Banana	1/2 small
Berries: boysenberries, blackberries, blueberries, raspberries	1/2 cup
Cantaloupe	1/4 (6-inch diameter)
Cherries	10 large
Dates	2
Figs (fresh)	1 large
Figs (dried)	1 small
Fruit cocktail (canned in juice)	1/2 cup
Fruit preserves and spreads (sugar free)	2 tablespoons

Fruit	Serving portion
Grapefruit	½ small
Grapefruit juice	½ cup
Grapes	12
Grape juice	¼ cup
Honeydew melon	⅛ (7-inch diameter)
Kiwi	1 medium
Mandarin oranges (canned)	¾ cup
Mango	½ small
Nectarine	1 small
Orange	1 small
Orange juice (any style)	½ cup
Papaya	¾ cup
Peach	1 medium
Pear	1 small
Persimmon	1 medium
Pineapple	½ cup
Pineapple juice	⅓ cup
Plums	2 medium
Prunes	2 medium
Prune juice	¼ cup
Raisins	2 tablespoons
Strawberries	¾ cup
Tangerine	1 large
Watermelon	1 cup

Complex Carbohydrates

Vary your choices of complex carbohydrates for the best results. Gluten-based cereals from whole wheat, rye, oats, and barley should be taken in moderation; healthy alternatives include brown rice, millet, and buckwheat groats. Whole unprocessed grains, enriched cereals, and legumes are good iron sources. The yellow-orange starchy vegetables (like sweet potatoes) are vitamin A powerhouses. All add dietary fiber to your diet. Specifically, you get about 2 grams of fiber per serving from whole-grain breads and crackers. Unrefined cereals and starchy vegetables provide about 3 grams of fiber per serving. Dried peas, beans, and lentils average from 4 to 8 grams of fiber per serving.

All yellow and orange vegetables, such as carrots, squash, yams, and sweet potatoes, are good beta-carotene sources. In order to absorb the vitamin A in this preform, the body must first break down the beta-carotene from the plant tissue. These vegetables must be prepared in such a way that the cell membrane is ruptured. Mashing, steaming, and shredding are the best ways to ensure maximum absorption from the beta-carotene-rich vegetables. Three or more servings per day are suggested.

Starchy Vegetables	Serving portion
Chestnuts, roasted	4 large or 6 small
Corn (on the cob)	1 (4 inches long)
Corn (cooked)	⅓ cup
Parsnips	1 small
Peas (fresh)	¾ cup
Potatoes (sweet, yam)	¼ cup
Potatoes, white (baked or boiled)	1 small
Potatoes, white (mashed)	½ cup

Starchy Vegetables	Serving portion
Pumpkin	¾ cup
Rutabaga	1 small
Squash (winter, acorn, butternut, buttercup)	½ cup
Succotash	½ cup

Breads

Bagel, whole-wheat	½ small
Bread, rye, pumpernickel, whole-wheat (Healthseed Spelt, Sprouted 16 Grain and Seed Bread, Woman's Bread, Ezekiel 4:9)	1 slice
Breadsticks	4 (7 inches long)
Bun, hamburger or hot dog	½
Croutons	½ cup
English muffin	½
Pancakes	2 (3-inch diameter)
Pita bread	½ (6-inch pocket)
Roll	1 (2-inch diameter)
Tortilla (Ezekiel 4:9)	1

Cereals and Grains

Barley (cooked)	½ cup
Bran flakes	½ cup
Bran (unprocessed rice or wheat)	⅓ cup
Buckwheat groats (kasha) (cooked)	⅓ cup
Cornmeal (cooked)	½ cup
Couscous	⅓ cup
Cream of rice (cooked)	½ cup
Grape-Nuts	¼ cup
Grits (cooked)	½ cup
Millet (cooked)	½ cup
Oatmeal	½ cup

Cereals and Grains	Serving portion
Popcorn	3 cups
Puffed rice, wheat, millet, or oats	1 ½ cups
Rice (brown, cooked)	⅓ cup
Rice (wild, cooked)	½ cup
Shredded wheat biscuit	1 large
Tapioca	2 tablespoons
Wheatena (cooked)	½ cup
Wheat germ	1 ounce or 3 tablespoons

Crackers

Matzoh, whole-wheat	½ (6 × 4 inches)
Pretzels, whole-grain	1 large
Rice wafers, brown rice (Westbrae)	4
Rye crispbread crackers (Wasa)	1 ½ crackers
Wheat crackers, whole-wheat (AkMak)	4 crackers
(Health Valley)	13 crackers

Flours

Arrowroot	2 tablespoons
Buckwheat	3 tablespoons
Cornmeal	3 tablespoons
Cornstarch	2 tablespoons
Potato flour	2½ tablespoons
Rice flour	3 tablespoons
Soya powder	3 tablespoons
Whole wheat	3 tablespoons

Legumes

Beans, dried (cooked) lima, navy, pinto, kidney, garbanzos, black	½ cup
Beans, baked plain	½ cup

Legumes	Serving portion
Lentils, dried (cooked)	½ cup
Peas, dried (cooked)	½ cup
Pasta	
Noodles, macaroni, spaghetti (cooked)	½ cup
Noodles, rice (cooked)	½ cup
Noodles, whole-wheat (cooked)	½ cup
Pasta, whole-wheat (cooked)	½ cup

Protein

Include at least two 4-ounce servings of lean beef, fish, poultry, and other foods high in protein three to four times per week. You may also include up to 2 eggs per day. Each food source is broken down to equal the equivalent of 1 ounce (cooked weight) of beef, fish, or poultry.

Remember, beef is graded in three categories. Select is the leanest grade, at 8 percent fat by weight, followed by choice at 11 percent fat, then prime at 14 percent fat. Make your choices from the select grade whenever possible.

Soy is are listed in the protein group because they are a popular vegetarian protein food. However, please consume soy in moderation—up to two times per week. Soy is an allergen for about 50 percent of my personal clients and nearly 30 percent of individuals nationwide. Soy-based products provide high amounts of the mineral copper, which my testing has shown to be connected to chronic fatigue, hormonal irregularities, panic attacks, and hair loss. Soy can also have a negative effect on thyroid function and the absorption of zinc and iron.

Shelton Farms, Harmony Farms, Foster Farms, and Young's Farm, commercial farm brands carried in natural food stores,

offer organically raised chickens and turkeys. Sources for
organic beef are Country B3R Meats (www.B3R.com) and
Coleman Natural Beef (www.colemannatural.com).

Food source	Serving portion
Dairy	
Swiss, mozzarella, mild cheddar, or Monterey Jack	1 ounce
Cottage cheese, 1 or 2 percent fat; Ricotta, part-skim or natural	2 ounces
Egg, free-range, omega-3	1
Fish and Seafood	
Salmon, halibut, perch, sole	1 ounce
Mussels, oysters, clams, shrimp, scallops	5 small
Lobster, calamari	1 ounce
Anchovies (well rinsed)	9 fillets
Sardines	3 medium
Canned salmon, tuna, crab	2 ounces
Meat and Poultry	
Poultry: white-meat turkey or chicken, no skin	1 ounce
Beef: lean—flank, top loin, ground tip, eye of round, sirloin, tenderloin	1 ounce
Lamb: leg, loin, rib	1 ounce
Veal: shoulder, rib, loin	1 ounce
Miso or tempeh	1 ounce

Dairy

Choose two servings a day from this group. If you have difficulty digesting milk sugar (lactose intolerance is especially
common among blacks, Mexicans, Asians, and Jews of Eastern

European descent), consuming dairy products in which the lactose has been converted into lactic acid may be helpful. Yogurt and other fermented dairy products like kefir, buttermilk, or acidophilus milk are usually better tolerated by the lactose intolerant, as is lactose-reduced milk. You can also purchase enzymes under the tradename Lact-Aid to use in regular milk. You may need calcium supplements, but remember that there are other dietary sources of calcium besides dairy products. Removing the inhibitors from your diet will help you make the most of the calcium you do get, whatever the source.

Dairy	Serving portion
Milk: buttermilk, acidophilus milk, goat's milk	1 cup
Yogurt: lowfat or full fat, plain; goat's milk yogurt, plain; kefir	1 cup
Whey protein (milk substitute)	2 heaping tablespoons

HOW TO HEAT

Stir-Sautéeing

Cook foods in small amounts of liquid or oil (water, peanut oil, macadamia oil, virgin olive oil, vegetable broth, or defatted chicken broth) at medium heat. Do not use polyunsaturated vegetable oils such as safflower or corn, which are extremely heat sensitive.

Steaming

Steaming preserves nutrients, color, and texture, and accentuates flavor while keeping in moisture. Cook over boiling water in a steamer pot, stainless-steel folding basket, or Chinese-style tiered bamboo steamer. The leftover liquid can be used for soups or stir-sautéeing.

When cooking highly concentrated carbohydrate foods such as sweet potatoes, steam instead of baking. The baking temperatures precipitate the natural sugar into a caramelized substance, changing the complex carbohydrate into a simple sugar.

Broiling

Cook in a broiler with overhead direct heat. Keep the oven door open. Nutrients are destroyed when the oven door is closed because the food dehydrates when surrounded by dry heat.

Toasting

Cook in the oven at baking temperatures below 300 degrees, ideally at 250 degrees. Seeds and nuts should be home-toasted, as low-level heating deactivates the enzyme inhibitors. Heating above 300 degrees, common in commercial roasting practices, changes the oil from the natural cis form to the damaged trans form.

Baking

Cook in covered dishes with a minimum of liquid to retain moistness.

Microwave

Microwave cooking heats the food by friction of the food's molecules. This is different from other cooking methods, in which the outside air surrounding the food must first be heated before the food begins to cook.

Cooking in a microwave does not make the food radioactive, despite the common misconception. Microwave cooking may even protect vitamins and minerals better than conventional methods, but care must be taken with certain foods. Because microwaves do not cook uniformly, rotating meats such as chicken and pork is necessary to protect against salmonella in the chicken and trichina in the pork.

Food prepared in a microwave may not be as visually appealing or appetizing because it does not brown during cooking. Convection microwave ovens or ovens with special browning features can achieve a more finished food look.

HOW NOT TO HEAT

Frying

Frying is all too common in coffee shops and restaurants, as well as in the preparation of popular snack foods such as doughnuts, potato chips, and many bakery products. Tasty as these foods are, overheating of polyunsaturated oils brings on oxidation of the oils and produces more free radicals than overheating of saturated fats; free radicals damage cells and may be one cause of common aging-related problems. These foods should carry the Surgeon General's warning!

When palm or coconut oil is used for frying, there are many fewer free radicals formed because these oils are saturated. Too much of the saturated oils presents another problem, though, because their presence can block the natural cis-linoleic acid from being transformed into the vital GLA. Plus, harmful toxins that have been associated with cancer are produced no matter what source of fat is used when it is heated at high temperatures (350 degrees) or reheated with the same oil source. When you do fry, do not reheat the oil; throw it out.

Browning, Charring, or Charcoal Grilling

The oxidative reaction of charcoal grilling (a combination of browning and charring) is toxic and can be carcinogenic. Further, food soaks up added chemicals, including benzopyrenes, from the charcoal briquettes. One piece of barbecued meat may be the carcinogenic equivalent of 60 cigarettes. Charcoal broiling should be avoided, but if you do grill, use a raised wire grill to lessen contact of the meat with the charcoal, cook 4–6 inches away from the heat source, cut off any burned, charred, or blackened portions of meat, or better yet, choose quick-cooking fish, rather than meat, to grill.

Gas grilling—with adequate ventilation—is acceptable if there is no sensitivity to the toxic by-products of gas combustion.

Pressure Cooking

Don't. The temperatures are too high and destroy vitamins. This method is suitable, however, for canning foods at home.

ELECTRIC VERSUS GAS?

For those who are environmentally sensitive, it is better to use electric rather than gas ranges and ovens for your cooking needs. The pilot lights and burners on gas ranges can release low levels of carbon monoxide and nitrous dioxide that often go undetected because they are invisible and odorless. Otherwise undiagnosable psychiatric conditions have even been traced to natural gas leakages. Symptoms such as dizziness, headache, chronic fatigue, confusion, insomnia, and respiratory problems can have their roots in unrecognized gas emissions.

If you suspect that you may be suffering from "indoor pollution," have your local gas company come to your house and check for a gas leak.

There are many other individuals who feel that the electromagnetic energy of food is disturbed with electric ranges and so prefer gas with proper ventilation.

POTS AND PANS TO CHOOSE

1. **Stainless steel**—heavy-gauge stainless-steel waterless cookware cooks food in a vacuum seal in its own juices. This is more expensive than the regular stainless, which is also recommended. Stainless steel, by the way, unless it is a high-gauge product, can be combined with an undesirable copper or aluminum base (see below).

2. **Enamel cookware.**

3. **Corning Ware.**

4. **Glass and Pyrex**—because glass and Pyrex let in light, they may allow small amounts of light-sensitive riboflavin to be depleted. Other nutrients are unaffected. Amber-tinted glass is now available and is a better choice than clear glass.

5. **Iron pots**—the extra iron picked up from cooking is good for you. When spaghetti sauce, for example, is cooked in iron pots, it contains six times more iron than when made in ceramic cookware.

Baking equipment should be heavy-duty tin or black steel. Glass, stainless-steel bowls, cling-free plastic wrap, or plastic bags (the kind used in the produce section of the supermarket) are best for food storage and freezing. There is also a hypoallergenic cellophane bag now available at health food stores for more sensitive individuals. The above-mentioned materials do not dissolve into the food.

WHAT NOT TO CHOOSE

1. **Aluminum cookware.** Aluminum-proof the kitchen—as I have indicated, aluminum hampers the body's utilization of calcium, magnesium, and phosphorus, as well as vitamin A. Impaired memory and motor coordination may be linked to systemic aluminum toxicity.

   Check all pots, pans, steamers, measuring cups, spoons, bread pans, and cookie sheets. These items can all be safely replaced by Pyrex or dairy tin (an old-fashioned baking material). An easy way to check for aluminum is with a small magnet; it will not stick to aluminum.

   No food or drink, especially tomato-based or other acidic foods, should be cooked in or covered with aluminum or aluminum foil. Instead of foil, use parchment paper in cooking and reheating. It is available in most health food stores and is excellent for retaining flavor because the food cooks in its own juice. Made from wood pulp, it is a healthy alternative to metals and plastics. Ideal for vegetables and fish (as New Orleans cooks have known for years), parchment paper can be used for baking and poaching. The food is placed on top of a moistened parchment sheet, then the corners are gathered up and tied securely.

2. **Avoid unlined copper pots and pans**—copper can con-
   taminate acidic food and destroy vitamin C; it is also
   antagonistic to zinc. Brass containers are usually made with
   copper, so do not store food in them.

3. **Replace or give a Clorox bath to wooden cutting and
   chopping boards**—bacteria can live in the cracks of
   wooden blocks. Use a Lucite chopping board, or give your
   wooden board a Clorox rinse (use approximately 10 drops
   of Clorox bleach to a quart of water).

4. **Throw out cracked dishes**—again, bacteria can live in the
   cracks of cups and plates. These bacteria will mix with hot
   beverages or foods, creating digestive problems.

JUST A NOTE ABOUT LIFE IN THE GREAT OUTDOORS

When camping out, remember to take extra care with certain
foods. Ground meat is more subject to oxidation than whole
meat. Cook it as soon as possible.

Do not drink water from streams and lakes, because many
are contaminated with a protozoa called *Giardia lamblia*, the
most frequent cause of waterborne illness in the country today. This amoebalike one-celled organism can cause chronic
diarrhea and has been implicated in chronic fatigue syndrome, allergy, and malabsorption. It makes its home in the
upper gastrointestinal tract and gallbladder. Boil all question-
able water for at least 10 minutes at a rolling boil.

CHAPTER ELEVEN

A Guide for Dining Out

A cheerful heart hath a continual feast.
—PROVERBS 15:15

Did you know that in the late 1990s, it was determined by the USDA that 57 percent of Americans ate out on any given day? Of those people, 32 percent ate something akin to a burger and fries. Gone are the days of the family eating a home-cooked, well-balanced meal at home. Based on eating trends in the 1990s, eating out has become more common than eating in.

There are some basic food considerations to keep in mind when dining out. First, look for foods that feature the essential or healthy fats. Choose cuisines that use olive oil (Italian, Greek, Spanish, and in some cases, French). Some Japanese and Chinese dishes use either sesame or peanut oil for stir-frying. Even carefully chosen Mexican dishes are good nutritional choices; guacamole features the heart-protecting monounsaturated fats and can be used as an appetizer or topping, instead of sour cream or cheese.

Keep in mind that the majority of undesirable saturated and damaged fats, salts, and sugars are hidden in sauces and dressings. Ask for all sauces and dressings on the side. Dip your fork into the dressing before it goes into the salad to control total fat intake. Enjoy creamed sauces in moderation or pass over them in favor of dishes with wine-based sauces, such as coq au vin (chicken cooked in red wine sauce). Likewise, try to avoid creamed soups in favor of tomato-based, vegetable, or bean soups. Choose Manhattan instead of New England clam chowder, for example.

Avoid unwanted fats by ordering seafood, beef, and poultry broiled, poached, or grilled, and ask that no fat be used for basting during cooking.

Eliminate tuna, shrimp, chicken, and egg salads from your diet when eating out because they are usually loaded with too much commercial mayonnaise. Mayonnaise is actually a processed food containing heat-treated and partially hydrogenated soybean oil. At home you can use brands such as Spectrum mayonnaise or make it yourself from expeller-pressed oils.

When eating out, watch salad bar offerings like cole slaw, potato salad, and pasta salads, which can also be loaded with mayonnaise. Instead of dips made with mayonnaise (or sour cream), order guacamole, hummus (chickpea spread), or Mexican salsas. "Lemonize" these dips by lacing them with lemon or lime to further cut the amount of fat. For sandwiches, substitute mustard and add healthy, tasty items like lettuce, tomato, and onion.

In the bread department, best bets are whole-wheat, rye, or sourdough bread and rolls. Prebuttered rolls, toast, and croissants (at 2–3 teaspoons of baked-in butter per croissant) should be limited. While butter is a much more healthful choice than margarine, it still should be taken in moderation. One to three pats of butter per meal, on a baked potato, for example, is usually reasonable. Eliminate margarine entirely. Ordering onions, chives, leeks, and garlic with meals adds both taste and fat-fighting benefits.

You should basically avoid all fried foods, especially those with breading; the bread coating increases fat absorption, giving breaded fried chicken and fish a higher fat content than a juicy hamburger. Other fried no-nos include tortilla chips, potato skins, Chinese egg or spring rolls, shrimp or vegetable tempura, and french fries. At home, you can make your own fries by coating sliced potatoes with a drop of olive oil and then baking them in the oven.

Starting your meal with a cup or bowl of hot soup can actually help you cut calories while adding valuable nutrients. A study at St. Luke's–Roosevelt Hospital, New York, found that when a group started its meal with soup, for every calorie the soup added to the meals, two fewer calories were eaten with the entree. The researchers believe that the soup moves into the small intestine more quickly than solid food, so triggers satiety receptors faster. See below for some nutritious choices.

A NOTE ABOUT SEAFOOD

With the growing pollution of our rivers, streams, and oceans, there is some cause for concern about the fish and seafood that inhabit these waters. Not enough is known about the long-term effects of consuming contaminated fish and shellfish. At this time, however, experts agree with Clyde Dawe, M.D., a Harvard Medical School researcher who has studied the problem for more than 25 years, "People should not be so scared that they stop eating fish."[1]

However, it does pay to be a wise consumer of fish and shellfish. The experts recommend the following:

• Eat a variety of seafood to lessen your risk of contamination from any one source.

• Cook seafood thoroughly. Avoid all raw fish or shellfish.

• Ask about the source of the fish you purchase. Most fish is caught beyond three miles from the coastal waters, safer in terms of contaminants than inland sources.

• Avoid eating fish skin and trim visible fat, both of which may contain higher levels of contaminants.

• Younger, smaller fish are more likely to contain fewer contaminants than older, larger fish.

• Avoid eating the tomalley in lobster or the "mustard" in blue crab. This organ concentrates the contaminants within the seafood.

• Women of childbearing age should limit consumption of fatty fish. Bluefish, salmon, striped bass, swordfish, and freshwater fish, especially from the Great Lakes, can contain high levels of PCBs, which have been shown to be harmful to fetuses and infant development.

• According to an FDA advisory, pregnant women and women considering pregnancy should not eat shark, swordfish, king mackerel, or tilefish because they could contain enough mercury to harm an unborn infant's nervous system. The advisory says that nursing women should also avoid those species of fish, which tend to live longer and so have higher mercury concentrations in their tissues.

A toll-free national hotline has been established for individuals who want more information about seafood safety and
preparation. Available weekdays from 9 A.M. to 5 P.M. Eastern
Standard Time, the hotline number is 1-800-EAT-FISH.

ALL-AMERICAN EATING

In standard restaurants and coffee shops, there are many options for nutritious meals. Consider oatmeal or poached or
boiled eggs for breakfast. You can add a couple of slices of un-
buttered whole-grain toast. For lunch, soup and salad are still
good mainstays. Hearty lentil, split pea, mushroom barley,
black bean, and minestrone are satisfying and high in iron,
B vitamins, and fiber. If necessary, you can skim the excess fat
by dropping an ice cube into the soup, then skimming both
the melting ice and fat that has been pulled to the surface. In
hot weather, cold cucumber-yogurt or gazpacho soup fills the
bill and provides valuable calcium. Main course salads such as
Niçoise, Greek, or Waldorf (lemonize this one well because of
the mayonnaise) are good luncheon fare, as are a chef's salad
without the ham or a Cobb salad without the bacon and with
less cheese.

Dinners can be built around any baked, broiled, grilled, or
poached fish, seafood, chicken, beef, or lamb dish with steamed
vegetables and salad. Healthful herbs like parsley and chives
are often available for cooking or edible garnish. Since lun-
cheons and dinners are nutritionally interchangeable, you can
vary your meal's offerings, depending on your schedule.

Even fast-food restaurants offer some fairly nutritionally
sound yet quick and convenient foods. Wendy's bowl of chili

is one of the lower-fat items on a fast-food menu with 28 percent of its calories from fat. A regular McDonald's hamburger without sauces and toppings is only 31 percent fat (add all the trimmings for a Big Mac and you have over 50 percent of the calories from fat!).

What about beverages with meals? Bottled mineral water or seltzer, including the newer fruit-flavored sparkling waters, is a cool, bubbling alternative to the calcium-leaching regular and diet soft drinks. Fruit juices are widely available in most restaurants and can easily be diluted to 50 percent juice with the addition of water or sparkling water. Remember also that coffee or tea with a meal can inhibit iron absorption, and coffee increases calcium excretion. (If you cannot give up your coffee, at least save it for between meals when it is less harmful to your calcium and iron.) Steer clear of commercial iced tea mixes, although herbal teas are acceptable, unless candida is a problem, in which case avoid all teas. Many restaurants keep a selection on hand, or take your favorite herbal blends wherever you go.

ETHNIC EATING ADVANTAGES

Foreign cuisines provide many healthy and delicious eating options. Italian, Chinese, Mexican, French, and Japanese are America's current favorites, followed by Middle Eastern, Indian, and Thai. Trendy restaurants featuring Cajun and Creole cuisines are popping up all over the country.

Here's how you can get the most nutritional mileage from each one.

Italian

Make complex carbohydrates in the form of pasta or beans the highlight of your dinner. Pasta primavera (pasta with vegetables) or pasta with pesto (basil, garlic, olive oil, Parmesan, and pine nuts) or even linguine with red clam or mussel sauce are wonderful meal choices. Risotto (rice) and polenta (cornmeal) may be featured in northern Italian cuisine.

A hearty bowl of minestrone or pasta/bean/vegetable soup can serve as a one-dish meal all by itself. Veal dishes, like veal marsala, piccata, or scallopini, are often deliciously prepared at Italian restaurants. Simply add a green salad and sautéed vegetables. (Fresh vegetables usually abound in Italian cooking— sautéed peppers, zucchini, spinach, escarole, cauliflower, and eggplant.)

Escarole in chicken broth is my personal favorite as an appetizer. I also enjoy steamed or plain baked artichokes. No matter what I order, I always have several fresh lemon slices on the side to help emulsify any excess oil from whatever the source.

To avoid carbohydrate overload or gluten problems, skip the bread if you are having pasta.

Chinese

First, request that no monosodium glutamate (MSG), sugar, salt, or soy sauce be added during cooking. If you suspect an allergy to corn, also request that cornstarch be omitted. If peanut oil is used for cooking, choose light stir-fries of beef (flank steak is usually used), chicken, seafood, or tofu (bean curd), mixed with vegetables like bean sprouts, onions, water chestnuts, broccoli, scallions, bamboo shoots, and calcium-rich bok choy. Cellophane noodles made of rice or mung beans go well with small amounts of chicken, beef, tofu, or seafood in lo mein dishes (these are not choices for candida sufferers). Buddha's Delight, a vegetarian feast of mixed vegetables and noodles, is a favorite. I love eggplant in garlic sauce.

In general, Cantonese, which tends to have light sauces and crisp cooked vegetables, is a better choice than the heavier Szechuan or Hunan styles.

A word of caution: avoid oyster and black bean sauces, which are highly salted. Ask for hot mustard, minced garlic, scallions, and some Chinese five-spice powder from the kitchen instead.

Mexican

Tasty first courses include black bean soup, gazpacho, and guacamole seasoned with lots of fresh lemon and lime juice. Choose from entrees like chicken fajitas and chicken or shrimp with rice. Tortillas, which should be corn rather than flour because less lard is used, can be steamed rather than fried; even quesadillas can be griddle-toasted instead of fried. Bean, chicken, or seafood burritos or enchiladas (minus the cheese), served with a dollop of sour cream and topped with lively salsa, are good options. Vegetables like chilies, squash blossoms, jicama, and chayote play a leading role in fine Mexican cuisine. Refried beans, however, are usually off limits because they are frequently made with lard.

French

France's cuisine boasts a wide variety of broiled, poached, and steamed foods. A selection such as fish en papillote, a traditional French favorite, is a delicious way to cook fish with herbs in its own juices. Other dishes such as bouillabaisse, coq au vin, poached salmon (without a heavy butter or cream sauce), and poulet aux fines herbes (roast chicken with herbs) are also suggested. Steamed mussels and that robust vegetable casserole, ratatouille, are also healthful menu selections.

Japanese

As with traditional Chinese fare, watch out for soy sauce. "Light" Japanese soy sauce is no less salty than regular soy sauce, just lighter in color. Also stay clear of teriyaki dishes (the sauce is a blend of soy sauce, sake, and sugar) as well as miso, a fermented soybean paste. Not only are these also high in salt, but all three items encourage yeast growth.

Japanese food has become synonymous with sushi. Raw fish is not recommended, no matter how meticulously prepared, because of the increasing levels of parasites and contamination being found in seafood at this time. However, sushi with avocado, cucumber, smoked salmon, or cooked crab or shrimp can be eaten safely. The green horseradish (wasabi) and pickled gingerroot accompaniments are strongly flavored condiments that are healthful additions. Noodle dishes with vegetables and chicken, steamed red snapper, grilled salmon or flounder are excellent selections. Calcium- and iron-rich hijiki is often braised in combination with mushrooms and carrots. Tofu-based soups made with kombu or wakame are safe bets (see Chapter Nine for more on versatile, healthful sea vegetables).

Other Ethnic and Regional Cuisines

In Middle Eastern and Greek restaurants, dips like hummus (garbanzo bean paté with sesame paste, garlic, and lemon) and babaghanoush (eggplant paté with sesame paste, garlic, and lemon) are served with pita bread. Used as an appetizer or salad dressing, these dips are good alone or cut with tzatziki (yogurt and cucumber). Side dishes of couscous (wheat-based pilafs) and rice-based pilafs can be found on the menu, along with tabouli, a grain salad of bulgur wheat, parsley, onion, tomatoes, mint, olive oil, and lemon. Greek salads or other feta cheese salads are wise nutrition choices. Shish kabob with meat and vegetables is also healthful.

If you go Indian, the pilafs and biryanis (rice-based dishes) and dals (bean-based dishes) are delicious. The sweeter, nutty-flavored basmati rice may be on the menu. Chicken and lamb can be cooked tandoori style in a clay oven, which seems to retain sufficient moisture, unlike broiling meat in a regular closed oven. Chicken or lamb korma with coriander and yogurt sauce makes a satisfying entree. If you like spicy-hot food, then vegetable and chicken curries will suit your taste. The dalia salad (bulgur, snow peas, and tomato with olive oil) is the Indian version of tabouli. Yogurt sauces and vegetables cooked in ghee (clarified butter) are permissible in small amounts. Pappadams (lentil wafers) are also permitted if they are baked, not fried. Chapatis and nan (garlic- or onion-accented bread) should also be baked, not fried. One item to watch is coconut, in the form of shredded garnish, oil, or milk used in cooking. These are high in saturated fat, the wrong kind of fat.

If you have discovered the unusual tastes of Cajun and Creole cooking, keep in mind that the simpler the better. Blackened redfish (minus the butter), shrimp or crab boil, chicken gumbo, shrimp creole, and seafood jambalaya (without the salt pork for sautéeing and ham and sausage for seasoning) fall within my guidelines.

IN THE AIR

Keep in mind that in these post-9/11 days, many airlines no longer offer meals. But for those that do, many are able to accommodate special diets if they are notified at least 24 hours ahead of schedule. Vegetarian, low-sodium, or American Heart Association diet–based meals are usually available and, in some cases, are tastier than the standard fare, as well as healthier.

ON THE HIGH SEAS

Cruises are known for a number of things, one of which is the lavishness of their cuisine. If you are not careful, eating can become a full-time occupation on board, from early morning until late into the night. However, as with some of the airlines, you can request special diet menus if you notify the cruise line at least 24 hours before sailing. In addition, some cruise lines are preparing menu items more in line with the American Heart Association dietary guidelines.

As always, broiled, baked, or poached meats, poultry, and fish, accompanied by steamed vegetables and a fresh, green leafy salad, are healthful. Find an active partner and swim, walk around deck, attend lectures, or read instead of succumbing to the desserts and snacks constantly available. A cruise, like any other vacation, can send you back to your daily existence refreshed and invigorated by the change of scene and pace; it need not send you back with candida, nutrient deficiencies, excess weight, dry skin and hair, and lowered immunity.

CHAPTER TWELVE

Super Foods for Super Women

We may live without poetry, music and art
We may live without conscience and live without heart
We may live without friends
We may live without books
But civilized man cannot live without cooks.

—ATHENAEUS, GREEK WRITER

Super Nutrition for Women has presented the most current information about the very special needs of a woman's body. Armed with your new knowledge, you have the best opportunity to make responsible choices about the food you will eat and how you will prepare it.

The key is to become an active "chooser," an active participant in life—rather than just a spectator. You can choose to create health or disease tomorrow by the living habits you practice today. Knowing that you can make a difference in your own health is the first step.

A WOMAN'S MENU PLANNER AND RECIPE GUIDE

A well-prepared dish, according to an old Chinese saying, should appeal to the eye by its coloring, the nose by its aroma, the ears by its sound (crunch), and the mouth by its taste. We might add that for women who are concerned about health, a well-prepared dish should also contain high-quality protein, complex carbohydrates, essential fatty acids, and vitamins, as well as absorbable minerals such as calcium, iron, and other trace elements.

The following week-long menu plan and sample recipes show you how easy it can be to whip up nourishing meals. To highlight the variety possible on the plan, I've used different ingredients each day. However, you may want to repeat menus so that you are not left with too many leftover ingredients. Freeze muffins and breads so they are available and fresh when you want them.

I have included name brands when particular brands provide higher mineral levels or other nutritional benefits over other brands for a given product.

The daily calcium and iron totals are included at the end of each day's menu plan. These nutrients were originally computed with the assistance of Computrition in Chatsworth, California, and *Agriculture Handbook* No. 8 from the USDA.

Items noted with an asterisk (*) appear in the recipe section that follows. You will also find several special recipes to introduce you to the flavor and versatility of mineral-packed sea vegetables.

Note: Choose from any of the following as beverages with your meals: herbal teas, mineral waters, or coffee substitute. Both regular tea and coffee inhibit calcium and iron absorption, so they should not be taken with meals.

Get ready, get set, enjoy.

DAY ONE

Breakfast 1 small orange
2 eggs, scrambled, with 1 ounce low-fat cheese
1 slice Healthseed Spelt toast with 1 tablespoon
  unsweetened apple butter
1 cup full-fat yogurt

Lunch Black Beans with Olives and Cumin*
4 ounces canned salmon with ½ tablespoon
  mayonnaise
2 sesame breadsticks

Snack 2 ounces puffed millet
1 small pear with 1 slice of Swiss cheese

Dinner Chopped parsley, tomato, and scallion with
  lemon juice dressing
4 ounces baked scrod with tarragon
½ cup steamed collards with 1 tablespoon
  sesame oil
1 small sweet potato

Snack ¾ cup prune juice

Total calcium: **1,354 mg**
Total iron: **16.5 mg**

DAY TWO

Breakfast 6 ounces of calcium-fortified orange juice
1 baked Ezekiel 4:9 tortilla with 1 ounce melted
cheddar cheese

Lunch ½ cup calcium-fortified tofu or 4 ounces of lean
beef, skinless poultry, or seafood
1 cup mushroom barley soup
1 slice Woman's Bread
1 small baked apple

Snack ½ cup low-fat or full-fat yogurt with
2 tablespoons ground flaxseed
4 halves dried apricots

Dinner 1 cup lentils with 1 teaspoon olive oil
1 cup steamed broccoli
¾ cup spaghetti squash with ½ cup marinara
sauce and ¼ cup grated mozzarella cheese

Snack ½ cup blueberries
1 slice cheddar cheese

Total calcium: **1,784 mg**
Total iron: **18.2 mg**

DAY THREE

Breakfast   1 small banana with ½ cup part-skim or natural
ricotta cheese
1 hard-cooked egg
2 heaping tablespoons of high protein (stevia-
based) whey powder mixed with ½ cup water

Lunch   1 cup steamed bok choy with red peppers
4 ounces baked garlic shrimp
½ cup brown rice with 1 tablespoon sesame oil
and 2 tablespoons grated Parmesan cheese
Carrot and celery sticks

Snack   1 ounce Essene bread
1 tablespoon organic peanut butter

Dinner   4 ounces broiled lamb chop with rosemary and
parsley
½ cup baked acorn squash with 1 teaspoon
butter
1 cup steamed green peas

Snack   ½ cup low-fat or full-fat yogurt
½ cup apple-cranberry sauce

Total calcium: **1,170 mg**
Total iron: **15 mg**

DAY FOUR

Breakfast 1 Fruity Fast Fizz* (with blueberries left from
Day Two)
2 tablespoons blackstrap molasses
4 whole-grain crackers

Lunch 4 ounces salmon with salsa
½ cup grated raw beet, cabbage, and daikon salad
with lemon juice dressing
1 cup cooked green beans
1 slice Woman's Bread toast with 1 teaspoon
butter

Snack 2 heaping tablespoons of high protein (stevia-
based) whey powder mixed with 1 cup water
2 ounces puffed kashi

Dinner 4 ounces lean ground beef burger, broiled, with
sliced onions and parsley
Spinach salad with 1 ounce goat cheese,
crumbled, and 1 tablespoon flaxseed oil
dressing*
½ cup buckwheat groats
1 cup steamed zucchini and carrots

Snack 2 dates

Total calcium: **1,340 mg**
Total iron: **13.8 mg**

DAY FIVE

Breakfast   ½ small grapefruit
1 slice Healthseed Spelt bread with 2 tablespoons almond butter and 1 tablespoon unsweetened raspberry preserves

Lunch   4 ounces canned tuna with celery, bean sprouts, and water chestnuts mixed with 1 handful blue corn chips
½ cup unsweetened pineapple chunks with ½ cup low-fat or full-fat cottage cheese

Snack   1 cup low-fat or full-fat apple-cinnamon yogurt with 2 tablespoons ground flaxseed

Dinner   ¾ cup macaroni and cheese
Cole slaw
1 cup cooked green split peas

Snack   ½ cup unsweetened fruit cocktail

Total calcium: **1,983 mg**
Total iron: **15.3 mg**

DAY SIX

Breakfast   ½ cup calcium-fortified orange juice
½ cup amaranth flakes
2 heaping tablespoons high protein (stevia-
based) whey powder plus ½ cup water

Lunch   Sassy Sardine Spread* on an Ezekiel 4:9 tortilla
Celery, jicama, and cucumber rounds
1 cup cooked lima beans

Snack   ½ cup low-fat or full-fat plain yogurt
2 dried apricot halves

Dinner   1 cup yogurt and puréed cucumber soup with
dill
Tossed salad with 1 tablespoon flaxseed oil
dressing*
4 ounces shrimp with bean sprouts, bok choy,
and carrots

Snack   2 small plums

Total calcium: **1,263 mg**
Total iron: **15.6 mg**

DAY SEVEN

Brunch   ½ cup grapefruit juice
4 buckwheat pancakes with 8 tablespoons
yogurt topping mixed with 1½ tablespoon
blackstrap molasses

Snack   ½ cup ricotta cheese with 2 tablespoons toasted
ground flaxseed

Dinner   Spiced Beef with Wine, Ginger, and Garlic*
1 cup butternut squash
1 cup mixed stir-sautéed greens with
1 tablespoon sesame oil dressing

Snack   1 cup low-fat or full-fat yogurt
2 tablespoons raisins

Total calcium: **2,311 mg**
Total iron: **16.5 mg**

Sample Recipes

Flaxseed Salad Dressing

4 tablespoons flaxseed oil
3 tablespoons apple cider vinegar
3 tablespoons fresh lemon juice
Fresh dill and garlic to taste

Put all ingredients in a small covered jar and shake vigorously for 30 seconds.

Makes 4 servings.

Black Beans with Olives and Cumin

2 cups cooked black beans
2 scallions, finely chopped
4 large black olives, pitted and chopped
1 tablespoon virgin olive oil
4 tablespoons fresh lemon juice
1 teaspoon dried cumin
2 cloves garlic, mashed

Combine all ingredients in medium-sized bowl. Toss well. Can be served hot or cold as a side dish or as a salad on a bed of lettuce or mixed greens.

Serves 4   2.5 mg iron per serving

Fruity Fast Fizz

2 small ripe bananas
2 tablespoons high protein (stevia-based) whey powder
   mixed with 1 cup of water
¾ cup strawberries or ½ cup blueberries, blackberries,
   raspberries, or pitted cherries

Place all ingredients in food processor or blender. Blend until smooth.

Serves 2   201 mg calcium per serving

Sassy Sardine Spread

1 4-ounce can sardines with bones, drained and flaked
½ cup part-skim or full-fat ricotta cheese
½ cup green onions, finely chopped
1 teaspoon prepared white horseradish

Place sardines, cheese, green onions, and horseradish in bowl and mash together until well blended. Serve slightly chilled as an appetizer, light main dish, or snack with crackers or raw vegetables.

Serves 2   400 mg calcium per serving

Spiced Beef with Wine, Ginger, and Garlic

1 pound flank steak, all visible fat removed
¾ cup dry red wine
4 teaspoons low-sodium Worcestershire sauce (available in
    health food stores)
1 teaspoon powdered ginger
4 cloves garlic, mashed

Place flank steak in baking dish and cover with mixture of wine, Worcestershire sauce, ginger, and garlic. Marinate for at least 2 hours in refrigerator.

Preheat broiler. Broil about 8–9 minutes on each side until done to preference. Serve hot with salad and vegetable.

Serves 4   2.4 mg iron per serving

TIPS TO BOOST CALCIUM IN YOUR DIET

- Add 1 ounce crumbled feta cheese to the bottom of a bowl of soup. The cheesy flavor and billowing white swirls add pizzazz to any vegetable soup.

- Try 2 tablespoons prepared horseradish combined with ¼ cup cottage cheese and 2 tablespoons yogurt puréed in a blender for a quick sauce over steamed beets, rutabaga, or parsnips.

- When making soup stock, try to include the bones of chicken or beef to increase calcium content in the broth. One or 2 tablespoons of cider vinegar will help dissolve the calcium in these bones for better assimilation, without adding any vinegar taste.

- Choose dark leafy greens for your salads.

- A Caesar salad with extra cheese, broccoli-cheese quiche, or a nog made with whey protein, egg yolk, crushed fruit, and nuts will give you calcium and vitamins C and D in one dish.

- Choose sunflower seeds for a snack—1 ounce has three times the calcium, four times the protein, and nine times less sodium than 1 ounce of potato chips.

- Select herb teas that contain combinations of these calcium-rich herbs: parsley, kelp, burdock, borage, and chickweed, along with some of the more exotic ones like horsetail, Irish moss, capsicum, dulse, and comfrey.

- Use any of the following calcium-rich tidbits, alone or in combinations, to sprinkle over soups, salads, and casseroles or as snacks: toasted sesame seeds, sunflower seeds, soy granules, pistachio nuts or peanuts, parsley or red pepper flakes, kelp powder, horseradish, wheat bran or germ, dried lemon or orange peel. Sea vegetables like hijiki in soups and stew provide 14 times the calcium in a glass of milk.

- Remember that the nongluten grain quinoa has as much calcium as low-fat milk.

TIPS TO GET MORE IRON FROM YOUR MEALS

- Since vitamin C enhances iron absorption, select appetizers prior to an iron-rich meal from items such as the following: tomato juice or soup, orange juice, citrus fruit salad cup, cantaloupe slice, or tomato and lettuce with basil–safflower oil dressing.

- Stuffed green peppers, made with lean ground beef, combine a vitamin C–rich food with an iron-rich one. Serve with tomato sauce and sprinkle with parsley and you add even more vitamin C.

- Cooking foods in large amounts of water can leach the iron from them, so steam vegetables to save their iron value.

- Pumpkin and sesame seeds are an iron-rich snack or garnish.

- The traditional cereal, milk, and fruit breakfast can be an iron booster by selecting strawberries, grapefruit, cantaloupe, or orange to accompany an iron-rich cereal. Substitute whey protein mixed with water for the milk.

- Combine 1 tablespoon brewer's yeast with any of the following to make an iron-rich beverage: ½ cup tomato juice, or ½ cup orange juice. Note that some people do experience diarrhea or intestinal pain when first trying brewer's yeast, so begin with ¼ teaspoon and work up to a tablespoon gradually. Also, since yeast overgrowth can be a problem, use these mixtures only as an occasional menu item.

• With as much iron as two eggs, a tablespoon of blackstrap molasses can be a valuable food source, despite its sugar drawbacks (see Chapter Five). Blend to a frothy mixture with a cup of water mixed with 2 tablespoons high protein (stevia-based) whey powder or use it in place of jelly on a slice of Healthseed Spelt.

• The preservative EDTA decreases iron absorption by as much as 50 percent from a given meal. Watch processed food labels and avoid this preservative when eating iron-rich foods.

SEA VEGETABLE RECIPES

As I described in Chapter Nine, sea vegetables are a new and exciting way to get calcium, iron, and other nutrients women need. Agar agar, used instead of gelatin, has the added advantage of slowing down the absorption of sugar, avoiding the peaks and valleys of sugar consumption. Thus it is a perfect addition to mousses and puddings. Hijiki, wakame, arame, agar agar, kombu, and nori are available in natural or health food stores. General instructions for preparation are included in Chapter Nine. These recipes were created for me by natural foods cooking expert Eleonora Manzolini.

Molded Vegetable Gel

6 cups chicken or fish stock
5 tablespoons agar agar flakes
1 carrot, cut into ¼-inch slices
4 sprigs watercress
1 zucchini, cut into ¼-inch slices
½ cup arame, soaked in water for 15 minutes
½ cup corn kernels, boiled

Bring stock to a boil in soup pot. Sprinkle in agar agar flakes. Simmer until agar agar is dissolved, about 8–10 minutes. Arrange vegetables in a shallow 2-quart glass pan. Carefully pour liquid over vegetables. Chill until set.

Serves 4

Hijiki Noodles

1 pound whole-wheat noodles, cooked and drained
¼ package hijiki seaweed, soaked in water and rinsed
   thoroughly
½ cup grated carrots
½ cup chopped celery
½ cup fresh minced parsley
½ cup minced scallions
1 clove garlic, minced
6 tablespoons extra virgin olive oil, salt, pepper to taste

Combine vegetables and noodles. Toss with olive oil and seasonings. Let stand 30 minutes before serving.

Serves 6

Cucumber Wakame Salad

1 pound cucumbers, peeled and sliced
½ cup wakame seaweed, soaked in water for 15 minutes,
    drained, rinsed, and coarsely chopped
1 tomato, cut into wedges
2 scallions, finely chopped
2 tablespoons sesame oil
1 tablespoon rice vinegar
1 teaspoon tamari

Combine cucumbers, wakame, tomatoes, and scallions. Mix
the oil, vinegar, and tamari together. Toss the vegetable mixture with the oil mixture. Let stand 15 minutes before serving.

Serves 6

Carob Creme

4 cups unsweetened apple juice
5 tablespoons agar agar flakes
2 tablespoons carob powder
1 teaspoon vanilla extract
½ cup low-fat or full-fat yogurt

Heat apple juice in a small saucepan over low heat. Sprinkle in
agar agar and simmer until dissolved, about 8–10 minutes.
Add carob and vanilla extract. Mix well with whisk. Pour into
1-quart shallow glass dish and chill until firm. Put set gelatin
and yogurt in a blender or food processor and blend until
creamy. Pour into individual serving dishes and refrigerate a
few hours.

Serves 6

Lemon Mousse

6 cups unsweetened apple juice
1 teaspoon lemon zest
6 tablespoons agar agar flakes
Juice of 1 lemon
1 teaspoon vanilla extract
3 tablespoons tahini
6 lemon slices for garnish

In a saucepan, combine the apple juice, lemon zest, and agar agar. Bring to a boil and simmer until the agar agar is dissolved, about 8–10 minutes. Add lemon juice and vanilla extract. Remove from heat and let set. Blend with tahini until smooth. Pour into individual serving cups. Garnish with lemon slices.

Serves 6

Strawberry Delight

6 heaping tablespoons high protein (stevia-based) whey
    powder mixed with 3 cups of water
2¼ cups fresh strawberries, washed and hulled
¼ cup maple syrup
3 level tablespoons agar agar flakes
3 level teaspoons kudzu, diluted in 3 tablespoons cold water
¾ teaspoon vanilla extract
6 strawberries, sliced, for garnish
6 sprigs of fresh mint, for garnish

In a blender or food processor, blend milk and berries until smooth. Combine in a saucepan with maple syrup. Sprinkle in agar agar flakes and simmer 5–8 minutes, stirring occasionally. Add kudzu to pan while stirring until thickened. Remove from heat. Add vanilla extract. Divide into dessert cups and chill for 2 hours. Just before serving, garnish each with slices of strawberries and a sprig of fresh mint.

Serves 6

MORE WAYS TO FREE FOOD FROM FAT, SALT, AND SUGAR AT HOME

For those of you who want to keep your current dietary program but need to make some minor changes in food preparation techniques and choices to get the most nutritional benefit from your diet, consider the following transitional ideas:

- Defat soups, stews, and stocks by chilling until the fat congeals and solidifies, then scrape off the top layer before reheating.

- Broiling meats and poultry on a rack allows fat to drip off during cooking. Meatballs can be prepared this way so that the excess fat drips into the pan under the rack, not into your sauce.

- If Tex-Mex or southwestern cuisine is a family favorite, refried beans can be homemade without the lard and salt in commercial preparations. Simply rinse canned kidney beans and mash well with water, heat, and add hot spices like cayenne pepper, coriander, and cumin for flavor.

- Instead of frying tortillas for homemade enchiladas, dip them in tomato or enchilada sauce to soften them.

- For ethnic dishes usually requiring breading and frying, poach meat in wine, water, or broth, and then bake in a covered dish to retain moisture.

- To replace high-fat, high-salt sausage, use turkey or lean beef instead and add spices like garlic and fennel.

- Broccoli, zucchini, and spinach with part-skim mozzarella make great pizza toppings instead of pepperoni or sausage. Veggies on pizza is one way to get children to eat their vegetables. Clients who have had to eliminate cheese from their diets because of lactose intolerance or genuine choles-terol problems tell me that they have discovered that pizza with tomato sauce, herbs, and lots of vegetables (but no cheese) can be as good or better than the traditional kind.

- To cut back on sodium, stock up on ready-made no-salt sea-sonings, such as No-Salt Mrs. Dash, Bell's Poultry Seasoning, fines herbes, and Italian herbs.

- Experiment with do-it-yourself herbs and spices, wines, and vinegars. Go ethnic with Chinese (mixture of ginger, cori-ander, and cayenne), northern Italian (wine vinegar and garlic), Indian (cumin, turmeric, curry, and coriander), Greek (lemon and oregano, or tomatoes and cinnamon), and French (wine, tarragon, and garlic).

- A fruit glaze can be used to frost cakes. Apricot, peach, or strawberry preserves sweetened with powdered stevia or fruit juice can be melted in a small saucepan, then spread warm on the cake.

- Freeze fruit-flavored yogurt to make your own frozen yogurt.

- Try frozen bananas or grapes for a natural, cool dessert.

- Some people find chewing on a cinnamon stick helps them beat a sweet tooth.

- Instead of adding sweeteners to cereal grains, use aromatic crushed seeds like fennel, cardamom, anise, caraway, or coriander. One-half teaspoon ground anise or caraway seed adds a Scandinavian touch to cream of rye or rye berries cereal.

• Natural unsweetened applesauce is a good dessert choice. Mixed with 1 tablespoon raisins and a dash of cinnamon, it is a good snack or side dish.

• Lifestream Essene breads made from organically grown sprouts are delicious toasted in a pan in the oven. The natural sweetness from the sprouts will satisfy your sweet tooth. Plain or spread with natural apple butter, Lifestream breads make for a satisfying end of the meal.

TIPS TO ENHANCE FLAVOR

• Season after cooking for more flavor. Piping hot vegetables can be tossed or drizzled with herb mixtures and oil. Hazelnut oil adds a real gourmet touch to cooked green beans, Brussels sprouts, broccoli, and snow peas.

• One-half clove of well-minced garlic combined with 1 tablespoon of chopped parsley and onion goes a long way to perk up any hot vegetable combo—and may give added protection against yeast infections.

• Sauce up almost any dish with a lively salsa from south of the border. Combine 2 finely chopped medium tomatoes, ½ cup finely chopped scallions, and 2 tablespoons finely chopped fresh or canned green chilies or jalapeño peppers with 1 tablespoon red wine vinegar. Chill in the refrigerator before serving.

- Grilling vegetables provides a unique smoky flavor, which has made grilled vegetables so popular in the most trendy American restaurants. Just preheat your broiler for 15 minutes and glaze your favorite vegetables with olive, macadamia, or peanut oil. Cook for about 6 minutes, then turn them over and cook until tender.

- The flavor of millet is markedly increased when the grain is roasted, similar to kasha or buckwheat groats. Just pan-roast until the grain turns brown.

MAKING THE SWITCH:
HEALTHY RECIPE SUBSTITUTIONS

My clients who are the most successful in achieving long-term benefits from my recommendations are those who incorporate small changes into their everyday eating patterns. There are many tasty ways to cut out damaged (trans) fats, salt, sugar, refined carbohydrates, aluminum, and gluten from your recipes, so you can incorporate my recommendations without giving up flavor or your family's favorites. The following chart gives some tips for replacing recipe ingredients.

In Place of:	Use:
1 cup margarine, shortening, or butter for baking	¾ cup macadamia nut oil
1 tablespoon of margarine, cooking oil, or butter	3 tablespoons ground flaxseed. Your baked goods will brown more quickly with flax, so either shorten the baking time or lower oven temperature by 25 degrees F.
1 cup sour cream	1 cup low-fat or full-fat yogurt
1 tablespoon cream cheese	1 tablespoon kefir cheese
1 cup cow's milk	2 heaping tablespoons high-protein whey powder plus 1 cup filtered water
Cream in soups	⅓ cup pureed beets, potatoes, and carrots to 2 cups simmering soup
1 tablespoon sugar for cooking	½ tablespoon honey, molasses, or pure maple syrup; or 2 packets of powdered stevia
1 tablespoon cocoa	1 tablespoon carob powder
1 ounce or square baking chocolate	3 tablespoons carob powder plus 1 tablespoon water plus 1 tablespoon macadamia nut oil
2 tablespoons margarine mixed with 1 tablespoon flour for sauce and soup thickeners	2 tablespoons arrowroot or kudzu (found in health food stores). Arrowroot adds calcium to foods, whereas kudzu is high in iron. Or use egg yolks to thicken sauces.
1 cup whole grain flour	Take 2 tablespoons out of 1 cup of flour and replace it with 2 tablespoons of flax meal. Reduce the oil in the recipe by 2 teaspoons for every 2 tablespoons of the flax meal. Bake for a shorter time or lower the heat by 25 degrees F.
1 egg	1 omega-3-enriched egg

In Place of:	Use:
1 cup white rice	1 cup brown rice (increase cooking time by 20 minutes if cooked alone, 30 minutes if combined with other foods)
Baking powder, regular (contains aluminum)	Equal amount of aluminum-free baking powder, low-sodium and grain-free
Breading and frying	Poach in broth, water, or wine, and then bake in a covered dish to retain moisture
1 teaspoon salt during cooking	½ teaspoon kelp powder after cooking
Gelatin	Agar agar, a seaweed gelatin available in health food stores replaces animal-based gelatin. Agar agar provides added fiber and lubrication in the intestinal tract by absorbing moisture.

In closing, may I wish that all of you who have read this book and are applying its principles enjoy a lifetime of quality longevity. As my grandfather Aaron used to say, "May you live till 120!"

Selected References

BOOKS

Appleton, Nancy. *Lick the Sugar Habit*. Garden City Park, NY: Avery Publishing Group, 1988.

Atkins, Robert C., and Shirley Linde. *Dr. Atkins' Super-Energy Diet*. New York: Crown Publishers, 1977.

Burkitt, Denis. *Eat Right to Stay Healthy*. New York: Arco, 1979.

Coffey, Lynette. *Wheatless Cooking*. Berkeley, CA: Ten Speed Press, 1986.

Connolly, Pat, and Associates of the Price-Pottenger Nutrition Foundation. *The Candida Albicans Yeast-Free Cookbook*. New Canaan, CT: Keats Publishing, 1985.

Cooper, Kenneth H. *Controlling Cholesterol*. New York: Bantam Books, 1988.

————. *Preventing Osteoporosis*. New York: Bantam Books, 1989.

Crook, William G., M.D. *The Yeast Connection Handbook*. Jackson, TN: Professional Books, Inc., 1999.

Dalton, Katharina. *Once a Month*, 3rd rev. ed. Claremont, CA: Hunter House, 1987.

Eck, Paul C., and Larry Wilson. *Toxic Metals in Human Health and Disease*. Phoenix, AZ: The Eck Institute of Applied Nutrition and Bioenergetics, Ltd., 1989.

Edelstein, Barbara. *The Woman Doctor's Medical Guide for Women*. New York: Morrow, 1982.

Fardon, David F. *Osteoporosis, Your Head Start on the Prevention and Treatment of Brittle Bones*. New York: Macmillan, 1985.

Frederick, Carlton. *Carlton Frederick's Guide to Women's Nutrition*. New York: Putnam, 1988.

Fuchs, Nan Kathryn, Ph.D. *User's Guide to Calcium and Magnesium*. North Bergen, NJ: Basic Health Publications, Inc., 2002.

Gittleman, Ann Louise. *Ann Louise Gittleman's Guide to the 40/30/30 Phenomenon*. New York: McGraw-Hill, 2002.

Gittleman, Ann Louise. *Beyond Pritikin*. New York: Bantam Books, 1996.

Gittleman, Ann Louise. *Eat Fat, Lose Weight*. Lincolnwood, IL: Keats Publishing, 1999.

Gittleman, Ann Louise. *The Fat Flush Plan*. New York: McGraw-Hill, 2002.

Hausman, Patricia. *The Calcium Bible*. New York: Rawson Associates, 1985.

Hills, Hilda Cherry. *Good Food, Gluten Free*. New Canaan, CT: Keats Publishing, 1985.

Horrobin, David F. *Clinical Uses of Essential Fatty Acids*. Montreal: Eden Press, 1982.

Hunt, Douglas. *No More Cravings*. New York: Warner Books, 1987.

Hunter, Beatrice Trum. *Gluten Intolerance*. New Canaan, CT: Keats Publishing, 1987.

————. *The Sugar Trap and How to Avoid It*. Boston: Houghton Mifflin, 1982.

Kunin, Richard A. *Mega-Nutrition for Women*. New York: McGraw-Hill, 1983.

Lansky, Vicki. *The Taming of the C.A.N.D.Y. Monster*. New York: Bantam Books, 1982.

Lesser, Michael. *Nutrition and Vitamin Therapy*. New York: Grove Press, 1980.

Long, Patricia. *The Nutritional Ages of Women*. New York: Macmillan, 1986.

Lorenzani, Shirley S. *Candida: A Twentieth Century Disease*. New Canaan, CT: Keats Publishing, 1986.

Marks, Betty. *The High-Calcium, Low-Calorie Cookbook*. Chicago: Contemporary Books, 1987.

Niazi, S. K. *The Omega Connection*. Oakbrook, IL: Esquire Books, 1987.

Ojeda, Linda. *Exclusively Female. A Nutrition Guide for Better Menstrual Health*, 2nd edition. Claremont, CA: Hunter House, 1983.

Page, Melvin E., and H. Leon Abrams Jr. *Your Body Is Your Best Doctor*. New Canaan, CT: Keats Publishing, 1972.

Pfeiffer, Carl. Mental and Elemental Nutrients. New Canaan, CT: Keats Publishing, 1975.

Pinckney, Edward, and Cathey Pinckney. The Cholesterol Controversy. Los Angeles: Sherbourne Press, 1973.

Polivy, Janet, and P. Herman. Breaking the Diet Habit: The Natural Weight Alternative. New York: Basic Books, 1985.

Rawcliffe, Peter, and Ruth Rolph. The Gluten-Free Diet Book. Englewood Cliffs, NJ: Prentice-Hall, 1985.

Reading, Chris M., and Ross S. Meillon. Your Family Tree Connection. New Canaan, CT: Keats Publishing, 1988.

Reaven, Gerald, M.D. Syndrome X: Overcoming the Silent Killer That Can Give You a Heart Attack. New York: Simon and Schuster, 2000.

Reuben, Carolyn, and Joan Priestley. Essential Supplements for Women. New York: Perigee Books, 1989.

Rosenvold, Lloyd. The Gluten Connection. Hope, ID: Rosenvold Publications, 1988.

Seid, Roberta Pollack. Never Too Thin. Englewood Cliffs, NJ: Prentice-Hall, 1989.

Truss, C. Orian. The Missing Diagnosis. Birmingham, AL: C. Orian Truss, M.D., 1982.

U.S. Department of Agriculture. Composition of Foods, Fats and Oils, Raw, Processed, Prepared. USDA Agricultural Handbook No. 8–4, 1979.

———. Nationwide Food Consumption Survey. Continuing Survey of Food Intake by Individuals. NFCS, CSFII Report No. 86–1, 1986.

Wallach, Leah. Food Values: Calcium. New York: Harper and Row, 1989.

Whitlock, Evelyn P. The Calcium Plus Workbook. New Canaan, CT: Keats Publishing, 1988.

Yudkin, John. Sweet and Dangerous. New York: P. H. Wyden, 1972.

PERIODICALS

Abraham, Guy E., and Ruth E. Rumley. "The Role of Nutrition in the Management of the Premenstrual Tension Syndromes." Journal of Reproductive Medicine, vol. 32, no. 6, p. 405, June 1987.

Adler, Andrew J., Ruth Shainkin-Kestenbaum, and Geoffrey M.

Berlyne. "Aluminum Absorption and Intestinal Vitamin D Dependent Ca Binding Protein." Abstract, *Kidney International*, vol. 37, p. 471, 1990.

AHA. Science Advisory on Folic Acid, Homocysteine, and Atherosclerosis (July 3, 1996).

———. Science Advisory on New Evidence for Role of Homocysteine in Cardiovascular Disease (Sept. 1997).

———. Science Advisory: Homocyst(e)ine, Diet, and Cardiovascular Diseases, #71-0157. *Circulation* 1999;99:178–182.

Anderson, James W., Linda Story, Beverly Sieling, Wen-Ju Lin Chen, Marilyn S. Petro, and Jon Story. "Hypocholesterolemic Effects of Oat Bran or Bean Intake for Hypercholesterolemic Men." *American Journal of Clinical Nutrition*, vol. 40, p. 1146, 1984.

Bjorksten, J., L. Yaeger, T. Wallace, and coworkers. "Control of Aluminum Ingestion and Its Relation to Longevity." *International Journal for Vitamin A and Nutrition Research*, vol. 48, p. 462, 1988.

Bland, Jeffrey, Ph.D. "Break the Cycle of Monthly Discomfort." *Delicious*, March 1988.

———. "Building Stronger Bones." *Delicious*, July/August 1988.

———. "Candid Talk About Candida." *Delicious*, November/December 1988.

Brown, Michael H. "Here's the Beef: Fast Foods Are Hazardous to Your Health." *Science Digest*, April 1986.

Brownell, Kelly. "The Yo-Yo Trap." *American Health*, March 1988.

Bullen, Beverly A., Gary S. Skrinar, Inese Z. Beitins, Gretchen von Mering, Barry A. Turnbull, and Janet W. McArthur. "Induction of Menstrual Disorders by Strenuous Exercise in Untrained Women." *New England Journal of Medicine*, vol. 312, p. 1349, 1985.

"Can Aluminum Cause Alzheimer's?" *University of California, Berkeley Wellness Letter*, October 1986.

Carr, C. J., and Ralph Shangraw. "Nutritional and Pharmaceutical Aspects of Calcium Supplementation." *American Pharmacy*, February 1987.

Cooper, Kenneth H. "The Calcium Controversy." *Family Circle*, February 21, 1989.

Cowley, Geoffrey. "Cholesterol Confusion." *Newsweek*, September 18, 1989.

222

Curatolo, Peter W., and David Robertson. "Health Consequences of Caffeine." *Annals of Internal Medicine*, vol. 98, p. 641, 1983.

Dyerberg, J., H. O. Bang, E. Stoffersen, S. Moncada, and J. R. Vane. "Eicosapentaenoic Acid and Prevention of Thrombosis and Atherosclerosis?" *Lancet*, vol. 2, p. 117, 1978.

Eaton, S. Boyd, and Melvin Konner. "Paleolithic Nutrition." *New England Journal of Medicine*, vol. 312, p. 283, 1985.

Forgang, Isabel. "Heart Association Nutrition Expert Says Entire Generation May Be at Risk." *San Diego Union*, June 28, 1987.

Fox, Arnold. "Your Calcium Bank." *Let's Live*, May 1984.

Gaby, Alan R. "Cholesterol Confusion." *Pathways/DC Resources*, Spring 1985.

"The Golden Age of Natural Oils." *Delicious*, April 1988.

Grundy, Scott M. "Comparison of Monounsaturated Fatty Acids and Carbohydrates for Lowering Plasma Cholesterol." *New England Journal of Medicine*, vol. 314, p. 745, 1986.

Heaney, Robert, and Robert R. Recker. "Effects of Nitrogen Balance, Phosphorus, and Caffeine on Calcium Balance in Women." *Journal of Laboratory and Clinical Medicine*, vol. 99, p. 46, 1982.

Hepburn, Frank N., Jacob Exler, and John L. Weihrauch. "Provisional Tables on the Content of Omega-3 Fatty Acids and Other Fat Components of Selected Foods." *Journal of the American Dietetic Association*, vol. 86, p. 788, 1986.

Ince, Susan. "Indulgence and Denial." *Self*, March 1989.

Jibrin, Janice, and Randall Fuller. "The United Tastes of America." *Self*, March 1989.

Kaplan, Janice. "Exercising Bones." *Vogue*, March 1989.

Liebman, Bonnie. "Is Dieting a Losing Game?" *Nutrition Action Healthletter*, March 1987.

———. "The All-American Junk Food Diet." *Nutrition Action Healthletter*, May 1988.

McGrath, Mike. "Can Calcium Lower Blood Pressure?" *Prevention*, April 1988.

Mihalik, Maria. "Who Gets Anemia?" *Prevention*, November 1986.

Neilson, F. H., C. D. Hunt, L. M. Mullen, J. R. Hunt Jr. "Effect of Dietary Boron on Mineral, Estrogen and Testosterone Metabolism in Postmenopausal Women." *Applied Science of Experimental Biology*, vol. 1, pp. 394–397, 1987.

Nicar, Michael J., and Charles Y. C. Pak. "Calcium Bioavailability from Calcium Carbonate and Calcium Citrate." *Journal of Clinical Endocrinology and Metabolism*, vol. 61, p. 391, 1985.

Popkin, B. M., P. S. Haines, and K. C. Reidy. "Food Consumption Trends of U.S. Women: Patterns and Determinants Between 1977 and 1985." *American Journal of Clinical Nutrition*, vol. 49, p. 1307, 1989.

Prasad, Anada S., Donald Oberleas, K. Y. Kei, Kamran S. Moghissi, and Joanne C. Stryker. "Effects of Oral Contraceptive Agents on Nutrients: I. Minerals." *American Journal of Clinical Nutrition*, vol. 28, p. 377, 1975.

Quint, Laurie, and Bonnie Liebman. "Putting Calcium into Perspective." *Nutrition Action Healthletter*, June 1987.

Recker, Robert R. "Calcium Absorption and Achlorhydria." *New England Journal of Medicine*, vol. 313, p. 70, 1985.

Roblin, Andrew. "Clean Out Your Cholesterol." *Prevention*, October 1988.

————. "Splash on the Olive Oil and Cut Your Cholesterol." *Prevention*, January 1989.

Sorlie, Paul, Tavia Gordon, and William B. Kannel. "Body Build and Mortality: The Framingham Study." *Journal of the American Medical Association*, vol. 243, p. 1828, 1980.

Späetling, L., and G. Späetling. "Magnesium Supplementation in Pregnancy: A Double-Blind Study." *British Journal of Obstetrics and Gynecology*, vol. 95, p. 120, 1988.

Squires, Sally. "Being Alert to the Good Fish and the Bad." *Washington Post Health*, April 4, 1989.

"The Stanford University Guide to a Healthier Heart." *Prevention*, February 1986.

"Target Supplements." *Nutrition News*, vol. XXVI, no. 12, 2002.

Taubes, Gary. "What If It's All Been a Big Fat Lie?" *New York Times*, July 7, 2002.

Taylor, C. B., S. K. Peng, N. T. Werthessen, P. Tham, and K. T. Lee. "Spontaneously Occurring Angiotoxic Derivatives of Cholesterol." *American Journal of Clinical Nutrition*, vol. 32, p. 40, 1979.

Weinstock, Cheryl Platzman. "The 'Grazing' of America: A Guide to Healthy Snacking." *FDA Consumer*, March 1989.

Witkin, Steven S. "Defective Immune Responses in Patients with Recurrent Candidiasis." *Infections in Medicine*, May/June 1985.

WEBSITES

www.cdc.gov (Centers for Disease Control and Prevention)
www.niddk.nih.gov (National Institute of Diabetes and Digestive
   and Kidney Disorders)
www.fda.gov (U.S. Food and Drug Administration)
www.ag.state.mn.us (Fast Food Facts)

SUPER NUTRITION SUPPORT

On the Web:
www.annlouise.com

I cordially invite you to visit my website where you will find a continually updated schedule of my events, lectures, and radio and TV
appearances. In addition, please check out the forum on my site
where you can share your insights, concerns, ideas, and motiva-
tional tips with women all over the world. There is a special section
on the forum that is devoted to *Super Nutrition for Women*. With my interactive messaging board, I am sure you will find the support and
encouragement you are looking for that will help you to comply
with the program. You are also most warmly welcome to join me
and my Fat Flush Plan followers on our annual Cruise and Spa
Spectacular Weekend. Many of our participants have not been followers of the Fat Flush Plan per se and still have gained enormous
benefits (including weight loss and inch loss) by attending these
events. Check out our photo gallery and see what fun we have!

Notes

CHAPTER ONE

1. Wooley, S. C. "Feeling Fat in a Thin Society," *Glamour*, February 1984, p. 198.
2. Taubes, Gary. "What If It's All Been a Big Fat Lie?" *The New York Times*, Section 6, p. 22, July 7, 2002.

CHAPTER THREE

1. Mary Enig, *Know Your Fats: The Complete Primer for Understanding the Nutrition of Fats, Oils, and Cholesterol* (Silver Springs, MD: Bethesda Press, 2000), p. 85.
2. R. L. Atkinson, "CLA and Body Composition," *Advances in Conjugated Linoleic Acid Research,* vol. 1, 1999, pp. 350–2.
3. "Diabetes Trends in the U.S.: 1990–1998." *Diabetes Care*, September 2000; 23(9): 1278–83.
4. "Dietary fiber, glycemic load, and risk of non-insulin dependent diabetes mellitus in women, *JAMA*, 1997; 277(6): 472–77.

CHAPTER FOUR

1. Alan Gaby, M.D., "Cholesterol Confusion," *Pathways* (Washington, DC: D.C. Resources, 1989), p. 58.
2. C. B. Taylor et al., "Spontaneously Occurring Angiotoxic Derivatives of Cholesterol," *American Journal of Clinical Nutrition*, 1979, 32:40–42.
3. S. E. Langer, *Solved: The Riddle of Illness* (New Canaan, CT: Keats Publishing, 1984), p. 99.
4. *New England Journal of Medicine* 2002, Nov 14; 347(20): 1557–65.
5. "Cholesterol-Proofing Food," *American Health*, March 1989, p. 22; USDA data, 1999.
6. Robert C. Atkins and Shirley Linde, *Dr. Atkins' Super-Energy Diet* (New York: Crown, 1977), p. 230.
7. *Prevention*, November 1986, p. 106.

CHAPTER FIVE

1. Food and Drug Administration, "Final Rule" for Sucralose, 21 CFR Part 172, Docket No 87F-0086.

CHAPTER SIX

1. Shirley S. Lorenzani, Ph.D., *Candida: A Twentieth Century Disease* (New Canaan, CT: Keats Publishing, 1986), p. 26.
2. Cited in William G. Crook, M.D., *The Yeast Connection Handbook* (Jackson, TN: Professional Books, 1986), p. 315.
3. Lorenzani, p. 74.
4. G. S. Moore and R. D. Atkins, *Mycologia*, 1977, 69:341.
5. Cited in Crook, p. 275.

CHAPTER SEVEN

1. King, Patricia, "Rethinking Our Daily Bread," *The Los Angeles Times*, July 29, 2002.
2. Cited in: Beatrice Trum Hunter, *Gluten Intolerance* (New Canaan, CT: Keats Publishing, 1987), p. 12.

3. Hilda Cherry Hills, *Good Food, Gluten Free* (New Canaan, CT: Keats Publishing, 1986).

CHAPTER EIGHT

1. H. Spencer, et al., *Gastroenterology*, 1975, 68:990.
2. Evelyn Whitlock, M.D., *The Calcium Plus Workbook* (New Canaan, CT: Keats Publishing, 1988), p. 7.
3. Jeffrey Bland, "Building Stronger Bones," *Delicious*, July/August 1988, p. 12.
4. Neilson, F. H., C. D. Hunt, L. M. Mullen, J. R. Hunt, "Effect of Dietary Boron on Mineral, Estrogen and Testosterone Metabolism in Postmenopausal Women," *Applied Science of Experimental Biology*, vol. 1, 1987. 1:394–97.
5. Whitlock, p. 15.
6. *American Pharmacy*, February 1987, NS27(2):49.
7. *The New England Journal of Medicine*, 1985, 313:70.

CHAPTER NINE

1. Michael Lesser, M.D., *Nutrition and Vitamin Therapy* (New York: Grove Press, 1980), p. 108.
2. Richard Kunin, M.D., *Mega-Nutrition for Women* (New York: McGraw-Hill, 1983), p. 5.
3. L. Späetling and G. Späetling, "Magnesium Supplementation in Pregnancy: A Double-Blind Study," *British Journal of Obstetrics and Gynecology*, 1988, 95:120.
4. Guy E. Abraham and Ruth E. Rumley, "The Role of Nutrition in the Management of the Premenstrual Tension Syndromes," *Journal of Reproductive Medicine*, June 1987, 32(6):405.

CHAPTER ELEVEN

1. Quoted in "Being Alert to the Good Fish and Bad," *Washington Post Health*, April 4, 1989, p. 9.

Index

Page numbers of charts appear in italics.

osteoporosis (cont'd)
  risk factors, 128
  smoking and, 119–20
  sugar consumption and, 16,
      69
overweight women
  American, percentage, 4–5
  fat with sugar combination,
      and weight gain, 16, 77
  sugar consumption and, 16,
      69, 76–77
oxalic acid, 63, 115, 117, 119

pasta
  Glycemic Index score, 73
  serving portions and
      recommendations, 175
Perkins, David, 73
pesticides, 164–65
phosphorus, 135
  calcium-, ratio, 65, 116,
      117–18
  DRI of "bone builders," 129
  food sources, 130
  soft drinks and, 118
phytates, 49
  as calcium inhibitor, 23, 26,
      49, 115, 117, 119
  as iron inhibitor, 63
  zinc and, 139
PMS (premenstrual syndrome)
  A (Anxiety), 145
  C (Craving), 145
  as a deficiency disorder,
      143–46, 144, 145, 146
  D (Depression), 146
  dieting or unhealthy eating
      and, 2
  EFAs and, 10
  H (Heavy), 145
  magnesium for, 135

occurrence in American
    women, 143
  sugar consumption and, 16,
      69
Polivy, Janet, 19
portions, 166–77
  calcium source, 20
  complex carbohydrates, 20
  essential and healthy fats,
      167
  estimating, 18–19
  protein, 20
  serving size of fruits and
      vegetables, 20, 168
  soluble fiber, 20
potassium, PMS and, 144
poultry
  detoxifying, cleansing, 165
  irradiation, 166n.
  organic, 175
  serving portions and
      recommendations, 176
  thawing, 166n.
Practice of Aromatherapy, The
    (Valnet), 97
pregnancy and lactation
  FDA advisory on seafood, 187
  iron needs, 62–63, 137
  magnesium and, 136
  supplements and, 150
prescription drugs, common,
    effects on calcium and
    vitamin D, 121–22
Prevention magazine, 60
Pritikin, Nathan, 8, 31–32
Pritikin diet, 9, 14, 32, 33, 54
Pritikin Longevity Centers, 3,
      32, 33
prostaglandins, 10–11, 25, 40
  EFAs needed for, 40–41
  PMS and, 146

Recipe Index

About the Author

ANN LOUISE GITTLEMAN, Ph.D, C.N.S., author of the *New York Times* bestsellers *The Fat Flush Plan* and *Before the Change*, is an award-winning author of 20 books on contemporary health issues and a weight loss expert with over two decades of experience in public health and in private practice. Gittleman holds a Ph.D. in holistic nutrition, is a Certified Nutrition Specialist, and has a master's degree in nutrition education and a naturopathic degree in drugless healing. She has counseled men and women from all walks of life as well as radio and TV personalities, professional dance troupes, movie stars, producers, fashion designers, and athletic figures. *Self* magazine named Gittleman one of the top ten nutritionists in the country.

She has worked in both the public and private health sectors with thousands of clients over the years. Gittleman began her career as the Chief Nutritionist of the Pediatric Clinic at Bellevue Hospital in New York City. She also served as a bilingual nutritionist for the WIC (Women, Infants, and Children) Food Program at the Hill Health Center, a satellite clinic for Yale University in New Haven, Connecticut. Gittleman then went on to become the first director of nutrition at the world-renowned Pritikin Longevity Center in Santa Monica, California.

Gittleman's Fat Flush Plan lifestyle approach is the culmination of her own search for the ideal weight control system, her success with clients, and her discovery of the Five Hidden Weight Gain Factors that sabotage weight loss. "Most diets simply target one or two of these factors. Fat Flush identifies, addresses, and corrects each and every one of them."

Her in-depth knowledge of nutrition, breadth of experience, and insights have placed her at the top of her profession, with over 3.5 million books in print. She was the first nutritionist in the country to sound the alarm on the no- to low-fat diet mind-set in her book *Beyond Pritikin*. She introduced American women to the new term *perimenopause* in her groundbreaking book *Before the Change* and began talking about the connection between internal cleansing and beauty in her book *The Living Beauty Detox Program*.

Highly respected as a dynamic speaker and savvy media personality, Gittleman has been a frequent guest on radio and television for 20 years. She is a regular on nationally syndicated radio shows including National Public Radio as well as CBS and NBC affiliates. She has appeared on ABC's *The View*, *The Dr. Phil Show*, *Good Morning America*, PBS, MSNBC, Fox News, and *Good Day New York*, *Good Day Dallas*, *Good Day Atlanta*, and *AM Northwest*.

Countless major magazines and newspapers have quoted Gittleman or featured her work, including *Newsweek*, *Harper's*

Bazaar, *Self, Seventeen, Fitness, Cosmopolitan, Parade,* First for *Women, Woman's World,* The *New York Times,* and The *Los Angeles Times.* Gittleman is a featured columnist for the monthly magazine, *First For Women.*

She sits on the medical and editorial advisory boards of the American Menopause Foundation, the Health Sciences Institute, the Price Pottenger Foundation, *Taste of Life* magazine, Your Future Health, Inc., Healing Retreats and Spas, and *Total Health for Longevity* magazine.

She lives and works in the Inland Northwest.

For more information on Ann Louise Gittleman and her work, please visit www.annlouise.com.